AF886481

INTRODUCTION
TO
ISOPATHIC PRESCRIBING

INTRODUCTION
TO
ISOPATHIC PRESCRIBING

Peter J Twohig

Book 3 in the *Homoeopathy 2.0* Series

Warburton Press
Gosford NSW Australia

Introduction to Isopathic Prescribing
Book 3 in the Homoeopathy 2.0 series

Warburton Press
PO Box 9305
Wyoming NSW 2250 Australia

First Published 2021

ISBN 978-1-922470-04-1

Any views or advice in this book are, unless otherwise stated, the opinions of the author alone and should not be taken as a substitute for medical advice or treatment. If you choose to act or refrain from acting as a result of reliance on the material contained herein, neither the author not the publisher will be liable for any loss or damage of any nature occasioned to or suffered by any person as a result.

Cover illustration: Kate Twohig, *Bambusa Vulgaris*
Visit WildHomoeopathy.com

For Jason, Marcus and Andrew

Acknowledgements

I would like to acknowledge the late Alan Jones, master homoeopath, for introducing me to the principles of experimental homoeopathy, homoeopathic isotherapy, and vitalistic prescribing.

Also, I would like to thank my fabulous sister Kate for the beautiful cover illustration.

'In order to follow the path of knowledge, one has to be very imaginative. On the path of knowledge, nothing is as clear as we'd like it to be.'

Carlos Casteneda, *The wheel of time: The shamans of ancient Mexico, their thoughts about life, death and the universe*

Contents

Introduction to the series 1
Introduction 7

Part 1 Group Disease 15
1 Group disease theory 17

Part 2 Isopathic technology 37
2 Isopathic pharmacognosy 39
3 Isopathic pharmacodynamics 1-Modes of action 47
4 Isopathic pharmacodynamics 2-Remedial dynamics 59

Part 3 Resolution of group disease 77
5 Group disease treatment 79
6 Isopathic detoxification 93
7 Iatrogenic disorders 105
8 Isopathic potency selection 119

Part 4 Isoprophylaxis 133
9 Approach to prophylaxis 135
10 Prophylaxis in practice 145

Appendix - Theory of miasms 159

Glossary 167
Bibliography ??

Introduction to the series

I wrote this series of books because, as a student and practitioner of homoeopathy, and as a teacher, I was concerned at:

- the lack of soundness of homoeopathic theory, and the absence of a logical framework for discourse
- the modern disconnect between vitalism and homoeopathy, rendering the latter rootless
- the impossibility for homoeopathic technology to find a grounding in a referential philosophy
- the complete lack of understanding of isopathy, especially in relation to prophylaxis, detoxification, and so-called miasmic prescribing
- the number of my colleagues who had lost their way in cases, and *did not know where they had gone wrong*.

All of this made it pretty hard to explain to others, especially my students, how it worked. However, over the years, through case taking and observation of results, a rationale began to suggest itself to me. It was not a new one; in fact, it was a general validation of classical methodology, which I had always practised, for the simple reason that it worked.

I should explain at this point that I had been a psychic healer for longer than I had been a homoeopath. In fact, when I began healing, I did not know that homoeopathy existed. But as soon as I read the *Organon* I recognised homoeopathy to be a modality of vitalistic medicine, and adopted it as the major component of my general practice.

These days, though I still do not know just how homoeopathy works I'm satisfied that at least I have a handle on it, and that it can be elucidated. I feel obliged to share the results of my investigation in the hope that you will get an improved cure rate, as that is what we all want.

I must say that, though I was not surprised that my findings and formulations systematically validated the homoeopathic programme for the treatment of individuals, I *was* surprised to find that some of the important tacit assumptions of homoeopathy are not logically dependent on it.

I am alluding to isopathy in its several applications, especially homoeoprophylaxis, miasmic therapy, and detoxification, which together suggest a programme for the treatment of members of epidemic *groups*. The explication of these findings and their translation into practice will be the subject of the final book in the series.

What to expect

This three book series will:

- provide you with a deeper understanding of the philosophy of homoeopathy, thereby diminishing its mystique
- encourage you to adopt new ways of looking at clinical presentations while taking into consideration properly formulated homoeopathic theory
- reveal a multitude of ways to use potentialised medicines, both singly and in combination, to achieve results

- offer modern and common-sense formulations of homoeopathic concepts that can be used to adopt sound and logical prescribing habits
- demonstrate that using a variety of prescribing techniques and theories can result in a more confident clinical practice
- show how prescribing without the pressure of doubts and misconceptions can enliven and invigorate your homoeopathic career
- provide opportunities for practising an expanded range of medical skills
- contextualise your training and experience within a vitalistic framework and enable you to adopt a solid classical view
- provide an explanation as to why potencies behave the way they do, and how to use that knowledge in the clinic
- clarify vague concepts of potency selection, the constitutional remedies, detoxification, miasms, antidoting, aggravation, and prophylaxis, to name but a few
- deal with the issues of modern homoeopathy once and for all.

New concepts

With a view to simplifying the technology, and resolving the chief areas of confusion in homoeopathic philosophy and theory, I have introduced at appropriate junctures throughout the series a number of conceptual innovations and revisions. They consist of:

- the *Vitalistic Hypothesis* as a philosophical platform, and its development as a structure for homoeopathic discourse (Book 1)
- a vitalodynamic model of illness and cure (Book 1)
- a reconsideration of homoeopathic remedies as morphogenetic fields (Book 1)

- the (pharmacognostic) concept of a remedy's *intrinsic curative power* and the (pharmaceutical) idea of a medicine being possessed of *actual medical power* (Book 1)
- a pharmacodynamic model of *potentialisation*, the process by which the essential healing nature of a remedy is transformed into a curative power or esoteric medicine (Book 1; implementation in Books 2 & 3)
- the theoretical model of Expansive Modal Medicinal Action, to explain the numerous functional modes of homoeopathic medicines (Book 1; implementation in Books 2 & 3)
- a theorematic set - the nebula of existing homoeopathic principles (many contentious, some just plain muddy) newly systematised into one coherent body of theoretical knowledge, developed *ab initio vitalistic.* (In this I admit to being inspired to boldly go where no man has gone before by Harald Gaier,[1] whom I gratefully acknowledge.) (Book 1; implementation in Books 2 & 3)
- constitution - a revised and concise conceptualisation of the constitution, consistent with vitalo-homoeopathic development (Book 1; implementation in Books 2 & 3)
- the posological concept of the *healing gradient*, and its role in providing curative motive force (Book 1; implementation in Books 2 & 3)
- aggravation - exploration in the context of the vitalodynamic model, and solution (implementation in Book 2)
- Group Disease - an additional dimension to the acute/chronic/pseudo-chronic trilogy; in effect, a new general

---

[1] Gaier, Harald C. *Thorsons Encyclopaedic Dictionary of Homoeopathy: The Definitive Reference to All Aspects of Homoeopathy. Thorsons, An imprint of HarperCollins*Publishers, Hammersmith, London, 1991.

theory of disease, which facilitates resolution of certain prescribing problems, particularly in relation to so-called miasms, for which it is offered as a replacement (implementation in Book 3)
- foundational to the group disease concept, disease vectors as *morphogenetic fields*, or fields of resonance (implementation in Book 3)
- isopathy - redefinition, role and application (implementation in Book 3)
- homoeoprophylaxis - remedial exploration and demystification (implementation in Book 3).

Series composition
The Homoeopathy 2.0 series comprises three books:

- *Book 1 - A Vitalistic Approach to Homoeopathic Medicine* provides: an outline of the principles of vitalistic medicine as they relate to homoeopathy, a revised homoeopathic pharmacodynamic system, a revision, along classical lines, of homoeopathic theory, and an outline of its clinical applications.
- *Book 2 - Case Management as a Clinical Technology* provides: an implementation of the principles enunciated in Book 1 specially designed to achieve improved results in cases of chronic disease; case analysis, repertorising and potency and dosage selection advice from the first consultation to the final review; and strategies and therapeutic guidelines for the management of notoriously difficult classes of case.
- *Book 3 - Introduction to Isopathic Prescribing* provides: special protocols for treating certain categories of patients, e.g. group disease (classical: *miasm*), and those in need of detoxification or prophylaxis.

Beyond the technology

The series is more than just an explanation of the technology and how to use it. It is intended to:

- empower you to adopt new approaches to clinical technology designed to improve the rate of cure and amelioration
- provide practical solutions for case difficulties and prescription failure
- increase your prescribing confidence and ability
- encourage you to be creative in solving prescribing clinical problems
- help you to see that remedy finding and prescribing do not have to be difficult
- supply you with a raft of prescribing rationales and scenarios
- increase your rate of cure and amelioration.

Introduction

Preceding books in the series

Book 1

Book 1 in the Homoeopathy 2.0 series: *A Vitalistic Approach to Homoeopathic Medicine,* provided:

- a distillation of wisdom in the area of contemporary homoeopathic philosophy along vitalistic principles
- an introduction to a revised homoeopathic technological model along classical lines.

Also, with a view to simplifying the technology and resolving the chief areas of confusion in homoeopathic philosophy and theory, it introduced a number of conceptual innovations and revisions (see *Introduction to the series*).

Book 2

Book 2 in the series: *Case Management as a Clinical Technology,* provided:

- a detailed implementation of the principals enunciated in Book 1

- a guide to the vitalistic way of practising classical homoeopathic medicine in the clinic
- a revised homoeopathic technology specially designed to achieve improved results in cases of chronic disease
- case analysis, repertorising and potency and dosage advice, from the first consultation to the final review
- strategies and therapeutic guidelines for the management of notoriously difficult classes of case.

In particular, that book, with a view to simplifying the technology and resolving the chief areas of confusion in homoeopathic philosophy and theory, introduced a number of conceptual innovations and revisions:

- *the healing gradient* - its posological application in providing curative motive force (introduced in Book 1)
- *aggravation* - practical clinical solutions, especially in relation to the clinical review (introduced in Book 1)
- *group disease* - an introduction to the resolution of certain prescribing problems relating to it (introduced in Book 1; main treatment in Book 3)
- *group disease vectors* - though it has relevance to the current book, the main concept does its heavy lifting in Book 3 (introduced in Book 1).

Prefatory note to Book 3

In the introduction to the series, I wrote that one of my main concerns as a teacher was the lack of understanding of the role of homoeopathy in relation to the special areas of detoxification (sometimes called drainage), miasmic prescribing, and prophylaxis.

On contemplating this matter, I was lead to the conclusion that, while *all* of the principles of homoeopathy in relation to cure could be derived from observations of the action of the similimum, *none* of them could logically be derived from the success of treatment strategies designed to relieve problems in the special areas listed.

Further enquiry showed me that the common factor among patients in these areas was a strong correlation with epidemic groups. This is a correlation that respondents to the similimum do not possess, and which their cure is independent of.

The principles of homoeopathy as enunciated in Book 1, Chapter 12: *Principles of homoeopathic medicine*, therefore do not have application to the treatment of a certain set of individuals: the members of *pathological groups*. The treatment of such patients is always designed either to eliminate a disorder of a group (classical: *miasm*) or (in the case of prophylaxis) to assuage an *anticipated* group disease.

This book clarifies this matter and, except for the explication of the group disease concept, does not get theoretical. In that it demystifies all of the related matters, it is a landmark book.

Objectives of current book

The purpose of this book is to provide:

- a theory of group disease (including its displacement of miasmic theory)
- an introduction to the principles of isopathic technology using potentised remedies

- strategies and therapeutic guidelines for the management of detoxification
- strategies and therapeutic guidelines for the management of prophylaxis
- a set of non-curative protocols for treating certain categories of commonly seen disorders.

Technological innovations

As with Books 1 & 2, the current book implements technological innovations in certain areas:

- *Group disease*. This is an additional dimension to the acute/chronic/pseudo-chronic trilogy—in effect, a new general theory of disease. It facilitates resolution of certain prescribing problems, particularly in relation to so-called miasms, for which it is offered as a replacement.
- Foundational to the group disease concept, the concept of disease vectors as *morphogenetic fields*, or fields of resonance.
- *Isopathy*. Redefinition, role and application.
- *Homoeoprophylaxis*. Remedial exploration and demystification.

As with the first two books, this book assumes a knowledge of the general principles of homoeopathic philosophy and practice, though some of these principles have been restated using vitalistic terminology. It also assumes some knowledge of homoeopathic pharmacy, the Homoeopathic Repertory, and classical homoeopathic theory.

By following the protocols in the book the reader will be able to confidently prescribe to all cases in which the isopathic is the appropriate remedy.

Organisation of the book

Book 3 in the series is about the management of chronic disease which is impervious to the similimum: the type of disease which causes one to reach for a miasmic, or to consider drainage therapy (detoxification). Part 1 is an introduction to group disease theory, the foundation of isopathy, and an explanation of how it impinges on literally everything we observe in the clinic.

Part 2 provides a solid foundation in isopathic pharmacognosy and pharmacology, showing how isopathy works, and the various clinical results of prescribing isopathically.

Part 3 gives detailed guidelines for using isopathics to eliminate—or at least reduce—all forms of group disease and all forms of toxicity, especially if there is a history of substance abuse or iatrogenic disorders (often the case when there is a history of allopathic treatment). It also gives a rationale and protocol for the selection of isopathic potencies.

Part 4 is a treatment of prophylaxis, which is explicated for the first time.

There will also be a critique of classical miasm theory, which group disease theory supersedes.

Special features

Chapter outlines

Each chapter is preceded by a list of contents, to assist in previewing the sequence of topics.

Key concepts

Key distinctions, when they appear for the first time, are in bold type. They are also defined at the end of the chapter in which they first appear, and in the general glossary at the end of the book. Note that this is the series glossary, and is therefore the same for each book. Note also that key concepts reappear from time to time.

Example Sets

Sets of prescription examples have been included to help the reader understand the technology. The examples given should not be thought of as constituting advice—they serve merely as illuminations of the text. Similarly, it should not be assumed that the examples have been clinically proven. In clinical practice, each case must be treated on its individual merits.

Further reading lists

These appear at the end the book. These are not reference lists, and their contents may contrast with the author's views, sometimes to the point of disagreement. However, the author will have taken note of them. Their selective perusal may go some way towards assuaging the reader's temper. Because of the overlap in relevant material between books, the reading list is for the series as whole.

Abbreviations

Throughout the text, the following symbols and abbreviations are used:

<	(Causes) aggravation, worse for…
>	(Causes) amelioration, better for…
C, CH, CK	Centesimal scale of potency
LM, Q	50-millesimal (quinquagintamillesimal) scale of potency
M	Thousand (on the centesimal scale of potency)
ml	Millilitres

Ø	Mother tincture
X, D, DH	Decimal scale of potency

Also, in many tables remedy names appear in their commonly abbreviated style, e.g. *Sol-t-a* for Solanum Tuberosum Aegrotans.

Dosages

Unless otherwise specified, all dosages given in tables and example sets are understood to be ascending collective doses, e.g. involving plussing or the like.

Nomenclature

The *sources* of remedies are referred to in their common or, if they have one, their scientific style, e.g. silver nitrate, *Arnica montana* (Leopard's Bane), *Tuberculinum bovinum*.

Actual remedies, i.e. potential medicines, are, with a few exceptions, referred to by their Latin names, using initial capitals, e.g. Argentum Nitricum, Arnica Montana, Tuberculinum Bovinum.

Potentialised medicines (also referred to as simplexes) are referred to by their remedy names followed by their potencies, e.g. Argentum Nitricum 30C, Arnica Montana 10X, Tuberculinum Bovinum 10M.

Remedies collectively are referred to as the homoeopathic materia medica, whereas the homoeopathic pharmacopoeia (regardless of version) is referred to as the *Homoeopathic Materia Medica*, or simply, the *Materia Medica.*

The Index to the *Homoeopathic Materia Medica* is referred to as the Homoeopathic Repertory, or simply, the Repertory (regardless of version), and occasionally is uncapitalised, e.g. 'his repertory of choice'.

Male gender pronouns are preferred, to preserve textual elegance.

PART 1
GROUP DISEASE

1 Group disease theory

1 - GROUP DISEASE THEORY

INTRODUCTION
Morphic fields and morphic resonance
The centrality of the disturbance
THEORETICAL PERSPECTIVES
Group disease theory and miasm theory
Group disease theory and vitalistic theory
    Prototypical disease influence
Group disease theory and classical homoeopathic disease theory
Group disease theory and allopathic medicine
GENERAL THEORY - NOSOLOGY
Phenomenology
Dynamics
Sacrifice of the individual nature
    Individual awareness and the group
Aetiology
Typology
    Pathologies
    Remedies
    Technology
Scale
Vectors
CLASSIFICATION
Childhood group diseases
    Phenomenology
    Functionality
    Dynamics
    Suppression response

Environmental disorders
Toxicological disorders
Political suppression
Behavioural disorders
    Neurosis
    Triggers as group disease vectors
    Psychosis
RESOLUTION OF KNOWN PROBLEMS
General epidemic diseases
Systematic development of materia medica
A systematic programme of prophylaxis

Before discussing isopathy it is necessary to introduce the concept of group disease, to which it is the prime response.

INTRODUCTION

Consequent upon the determination of humans in every field of endeavour to impose ideal states, e.g. of balance, perfection, uniformity, conformity, behaviour etc, we are now faced with pandemics that reflect the loss of individuality and the growth of homogeneity: cancer, AIDS, influenza, depression, genetic disorders, and so on. In fact all disease, in that it results in immobility, pain and a lack of playful expression, may be seen as limiting the possibility of happiness, not only individually but socially.

The steady disappearance of our beautiful natural environment is just an extension of human group pathology. The vitalistic medical model is holonomic: it may begin with the individual, but it has ramifications throughout life on earth.

Nevertheless, the model as herein elucidated assumes that the individual when sick couldn't care less about the planet, and just wants to feel better. It is therefore pragmatic, and to that end, *individually* oriented.

In practice therefore, we *re-cognise* the pathophysiology, and treat the patient as a *member of a category, or group*. Moreover, in many cases we even know the identity of the associated pathogenic vector, which is a key element in isopathy.

Finally but crucially, it is important to realise that cure—or simple palliation—of the individual will resonate with the generative group, and weaken its infective potency.

Morphic fields and morphic resonance

Sheldrake's hypothesis of formative causation (see Book 1, Chapter 6) explains how species may learn and evolve through the interaction of *morphic fields*, by ***morphic resonance***.[2] The patient is, I assert, such a field, as are his disease and its solutions.

The centrality of the disturbance

When the patient's vital disturbance does not have its centre within his morphic field, it must be sought in a relationship bond with a higher-level, non-locational, morphogenetic field (in which case, we still speak of 'centrality' for want of a more serviceable notion) making it susceptible to a *non-similar remedy*. The remedy known as the isopathic is *also* a resonant morphogenetic field, one having resonance not with the patient but with the patient's higher-level morphogenetic disease field via a bond or path.

---

[2] Sheldrake, R. 2009, Morphic *resonance: the nature of formative causation,* 4th rev. and expanded U.S. edn, Park Street Press, Rochester, Vermont.

THEORETICAL PERSPECTIVES

Group disease theory and miasm theory

Book 1 of this series contained an explanation of the homoeopathic general theory of disease, namely that there is only one fundamental disease: disturbance of the vital force, a view that completely accords with the vitalistic view of disease. Early homoeopaths were of the view that this disturbance could have had only a single fundamental cause: the prototypical miasm, psora. However, this view is no longer supportable. (A brief analysis of miasm theory appears in the Appendix.)

Group disease theory and vitalistic theory

The vitalistic view expressed and validated throughout this series, is a *holistic* one, namely that disease is always and everywhere, and that any other view is materialistic, and therefore spurious. Naturally, however, in clinical practice it is convenient to take the historical view of the patient's presentation, i.e. what he says, what he points to, etc.

Group disease theory, like miasm theory, is not a theory of homoeopathic medicine per se but of *vitalistic* medicine. It differs fundamentally from miasm theory in the following ways:

- by allowing the individual to take responsibility for his health (and its absence)
- by not depending on physical concepts for validation, despite its frequent association with apparent physical disease vectors
- by being able to account for all illness
- by enabling every current group disease to be identified.

Prototypical disease influence

Group disease may be regarded as being the result of the presence on earth of a prototypical parasitical influence which causes the individual to experience delusion (that being the one symptom that *all* patients seem to exhibit). It is but a small step from delusion to the life of suffering born of ignorance. Susceptibility to disease types ensues.

Discussion of the prototypical influence is outside the scope of this book. However, throughout it there will be references to common disease vectors, many of which may be thought of as derivative.

Please note that this idea is *not* a version of the protomiasm, and is essentially more akin to the concept of evil.

Group disease theory and classical homoeopathic disease theory

There is no incompatibility between group disease theory and classical homoeopathy, because both are based on the principles of vitalistic medicine. However, group disease supersedes to some extent elements of each classical entity (and miasmic theory in its entirety) by requiring a reconsideration of just what it is to be diseased.

We might think of a group disease as a proving (of a specific toxic group influence) which may be dispelled (neutralised) by an identical influence in potency.

Group disease theory and allopathic medicine

Whereas in homoeopathic medicine the name of the patient's presentation may be thought of as the name of the remedy that might act curatively (or palliatively), e.g. Calcarea Carbonica, in *allopathic* medicine the name given to the patient's diagnosed syndrome, e.g. rheumatoid arthritis, is the name of (what is referred to in this book as) the *group disease.*

And just as a group disease as such cannot be cured by an allopath's use of **suppressive medication**, nor can it be cured by a *homoeopathic* remedy, though both might be used palliatively.

GENERAL THEORY - NOSOLOGY

A classical homoeopathic nosology was given in Chapter 6 of Book 1. It comprised chronic, pseudo-chronic and acute disease. For the purpose of comparison I have presented a picture of group disease using a similar analysis.

Phenomenology

The concept of group disease stems from the concept—fundamental to vitalistic medicine—that the vital force expresses itself in every way possible, one of those possibilities being the *group*. A group disease is defined as a disease of a group. Each distinct group disease may be identified aetiologically with a distinct group, and may be thought of as being related to the group psyche in the same way that the individual disease is related to the individual psyche.

Dynamics

The group may be thought of as constantly entraining susceptible recruits (i.e. those who resonate with it) and enrolling them by communicating its noxious influence. Inevitably, nodal crystals known as *group disease vectors* appear in infected individuals, signalling acceptance by the individual of contagion.

In this it differs from an individual disease, which results from the interaction of the life force with its altered terrain, namely the host organism. A group is a scalar phenomenon, being simply a manifestation of the life force in the human organism on a higher, e.g. social, scale.

Sacrifice of the individual nature

It should be obvious even to the casual observer that the individual cannot relate to the group on an equal basis, not only because the group is numerically superior (though numbers do have their own powers), but because it typically activates archetypal responses within the individual, and these archetypes are the true vectors of relationship. The individual in turn affects the group by presenting it with an essentially independent and mysterious element.

The group's response is always to sacrificially enrol the individual. That is why individuals with group diseases display common syndromes.

In order to survive, most individuals subscribe to many groups (the family being the first), often to their detriment. Groups enrol individuals with the same intent.

Individual awareness and the group

Note that the individual who *consciously* chooses to interact with a group may *not* be enrolled, and may be conductive to the group's vectors. This is one reason why the homoeopathic physician, who consciously submerges himself in the essence of the case, and its remedy candidates, remains safe.

Aetiology

In vitalistic medicine it makes no sense to enquire whether the individual disease preceded the group disease. We accept that certain weaknesses are endemic to humanity, and we accept also that every individual has the power to act egocentrically, and to thereby generate disease, which eventually radiates to relational spheres, where it influences others.

Homoeopathic technology enables the physician to treat the patient both as an individual and as a member of a group; that is the advantage of the distinction.

Nevertheless it is convenient to consider that, within his constitutional constraints, the individual will appear to make an endless stream of decisions, any or all of which could have social consequences.

What we observe in the study of group disease is the relationship between the individual and the group. The susceptible individual resonates with the group in some way, thus validating and strengthening it. Vectors may or may not be identified.

As a footnote, we observe that as a group disease matures, it manifests even higher-scale pathology, e.g. within a culture or people. An example would be the development of Marxism into postmodernism.

Typology

Group disease may be classified as:

- endemic
- epidemic
- political.

Pathologies

In the model as applied to epidemiology we see that (the vital force-fields of) susceptible individuals may be enrolled by group morphic fields by means of morphic resonance, resulting in the appearance in those individuals of typical (endemic and epidemic and political) forms of disease.

Remedies

When the model is applied to remedies, we see that it is through morphic resonance that the appearance of the *already similar* but unknown remedy is presenced by the homoeopath via an explication of the case. In this regard we may note that pharmacognostic invariability is the main feature of the *Materia Medica*.

Note also that it is the integrity of the original morphogenetic field that makes a remedy *proven once only* exert its force worldwide for every similar symptomatology and to never lose its healing potential.

Technology

Pharmacodynamic repeatability, i.e. invariable conformity of all aspects of potency therapy to vitalistic dicta, is a feature of every homoeopathic application (see also Book 1, Chapter 12), and ensures a high level of confidence in isotherepeutics.

Scale

It has been asserted that a group disease is an individual disease on a larger scale. What that means is that group disease is literally identifiable with individual disease: the difference is purely one of resolution due to magnitude. That is why a group disease on the scale of the individual may appear as a total symptom picture warranting a similimum that is *associated* with a group disease.

For example, the Medorrhinum group may show up in an individual patient as Cubeba Officinalis (the similimum), in which case the nosode (as isopathic) may only be needed to complete the case.

Thus, we do not observe the symptoms of the individual *as such* in the group, not because they are absent, but because we are not focused on the group qua patient. When, as they inevitably must, physicians begin to focus on the pathologies demonstrated by social groups: political movements, governments, malignant religions and cults, delusional ideologies, and so on, they will observe symptomatology in a familiar form.

Vectors

A **group disease vector** is any communicable noxious influence whose establishment in the individual signals acceptance of disease. It is important to note that the appearance of the vector merely signals acceptance of the morphogenetic field germ. In other words, it was not the vector which made the patient sick in the first place.

Nevertheless, it is often convenient to speak of disease vectors as if they are vehicles, since it allows us to speak of their elimination as signs of progressing therapy, though usually not complete cure itself. (See Example Set 1.1.)

Note that group disease vectors may also occupy and pass harmlessly though the bodies of healthy individuals, i.e. those in whom there is no susceptibility, or 'catch', though they may still be carriers.

A group disease vector may be potentised to form an isopathic that will have the effect of eliminating the vector itself. In the absence of a known vector, we can make a nosode from someone else who already has the disease.

Example Set 1.1 Group disease vectors

Possible vector	*Disease*	*Possible isopathic*	*Possible similimum*
Asbestos fragments	Asbestosis	Asbestos 6LM	Antimonium Tartaricum
Petrol fumes	Road rage	Petrol Fumes 6LM	Sulphuricum Acidum
Arsenic fumes	Arsenic poisoning	Arsenic 6LM	Hepar Sulphuricum
Alcohol	Alcoholism	Alcohol 6LM	Agaricus Muscarius
Fanatical religious speech	Religious fanaticism	Fanatical Religious Speech 100LM	Robinia Pseudocacia

Incidentally, the fact that contact with allopathic physicians routinely results in pathology suggests that those physicians may themselves be group disease vectors. (The expanding use of vitalistic—especially homoeopathic—medicine in society may currently be aggravating for that group, but amelioration will assuredly follow!)

CLASSIFICATION

While an endogenous disease may be exquisitely mysterious, making it impossible to divine its true origins, that is not the case with a group disease, which is far less opaque, especially when it is associated with a unique vector, or transmission signal, e.g. a virus.

Group diseases may be broadly classified according to their vectors as:

- infectious (including childhood)
- environmental
- toxicological
- political.

In practice they are all treated the same way. However, the distinctions may assist the prescriber to arrive at an isopathic. The following notes are merely designed to serve as examples, though they will have wide application.

Infectious diseases

Whereas adolescents share cultural diseases (mutually embarrassing), adults share national diseases (popularly uglifying), and the elderly share specific diseases, i.e. diseases caused by being born (auto-deformative), children have a propensity for group diseases of a social nature (innocently shared).

Although the following treatment is for childhood diseases, the principles of contraction are the same for adults who have been infected by disease.

Childhood group disease

Phenomenology

The childhood group diseases include those which are often referred to as the childhood acute miasms. An acute disease, i.e. one that is associated with a fresh vector, is explained in classical disease theory as an attempt by the vital force to eliminate a chronic miasm. However, the childhood diseases are not primarily attempts to throw off miasms; they are simply learning experiences for endemic group members.

Many individuals contract a series of infectious diseases during childhood, then go on to have normal lives, complete with occasional diseases, in spite of a minimum of suppression and a modicum of other experiential challenges—some more or less disastrous. They are evidence that the successful experience of acute disease and suffering is part and parcel of a healthy and often long life.

Functionality

Childhood is a time of development for the individual, no less so than for the immune system. It is the immune system that enables the individual to manage group disease vectors. A healthy immune system will respond to exposure by enabling the influence to be recorded, transformed harmlessly, and pass. The degree of the immune system's success is thus the measure of its conductivity. The slightest degree of resistance, on the other hand, causes symptoms to occur, worsen, or return as mutation.

Dynamics

Children are the best conductors of disease vectors, and are able to display highly dramatic syndromes which form well-defined diseases, whereas the adult, especially in later years, copes poorly with disease, and easily adopts a resistant state, due almost entirely to the *entertainment of delusion*, which is absent in the infant.

Consequently, the normal child is frequently ill. Provided that the child's immune system is healthy, and has not been corrupted, overloaded or destroyed, e.g. by exposure to noxious substances, vaccines, unnecessary suppressive medication, coercive influences, etc, his *entelechy* will develop a healthy discriminative ability, and in time conduct most disease vectors relatively easily.

Notwithstanding the forgoing comments, it is apparent that a great many children succumb to acute infectious disease in the absence of exogenous suppression. The inability of their DNA to code for the proteins and neurofunctional configurations necessary for conduction must be counted as a factor.

Suppression response

Note that the result of suppression of the individual human *in any way* invariably results in a kind of dehumanisation, in which the loss of individuality is replaced by a display of automaticity. We see this in educational institutions, prisons, mental hospitals, military forces, and the like.

Thus, it is not surprising that the suppression of the vital force of the infant, e.g. through **vaccination**, will often lead to *increased* automatic behavioural expression, e.g. autism. That is the mutational and metastatic response.

Environmental disorders

It is common for patients to present with environmental disorders, for example, the effects of air pollution, seasonal allergies and the effects of noise.

Usually they are treated homoeopathically, especially in cases of allergy. However, such treatment is always palliative at best. And eventually, hyposensitisation (an isopathic procedure) will be required (see Chapters 4 and 8 (for potency selection).

Toxicological disorders

By far the most common group diseases seen in the clinic are those relating to dangerous substances. If the patient's condition is socially acceptable, e.g. alcoholism, obesity, Type II diabetes, congestive heart failure, cancer, and so on, then the patient may not consider himself to be the subject of a group disease at all. He may, for example, have consulted you about something that may or may not be related, but which is simply inconvenient.

However, you will find that, if there is evidence of a vector, whether it is organic, chemical, then your primary task will be to address it, if possible.

Naturally, and especially in cases of addiction, symptomatic homoeopathic support will be necessary once treatment has begun.

Political suppression

Political ideology is the world's most widespread dangerous problem. It corrupts everywhere it inflicts itself, and always afflicts those who are not mindful of its presence. It is arguably the root of all suffering. Fortunately, its vectors—they are usually oral and literary—are easy to spot, sample, and potentise. Examples abound on the internet.

Behavioural disorders

I have included the following notes because I suspect that many emotional disorders are actually group diseases (though I know from experience that homoeopathics have a miraculous effect in acute cases). However, as group disorders, they are notoriously difficult to dispel.

Neurosis

A patient who emerges from adolescence somehow damaged by abuse, suppression and toxicity may be neurotic and a candidate for psychosis, depending on the circumstances, his constitution etc.

In a sense, therefore, neurosis of known aetiology is itself a group disease. When the ability to harmlessly experience emotions is lost, it is lost to *controlling group entities*: initially, the family, then wider institutions, and inevitably, society itself. The path back to wellness is only available to those who are able to rediscover that lost ability, and is so extremely difficult that few take it, and most go on living their life in delusion.

A small number of remedies (mentals, delusions, etc), suggest themselves in these cases. However, the problem is that the provers were not attuned to psychological matters.

One solution is to search the materia medica more diligently for rubrics; another is to get into an interpretive mode, though I would only recommend that approach to the mature practitioner, not least because of the ever-present risk of projection.

Triggers as group disease vectors

The vectors for neurosis appear for the most part to be triggers, especially verbal triggers, which stimulate emotional reactions more often—or more severely—than they can be managed, i.e. absorbed, integrated, processed or expressed by the organism. The neurosis remains in place and crystallises within the organism, initially as habit, then pathophysiologically.

The homoeopath recognises the signs of neurosis as persistent mental symptoms. But always remember that vectors are not causes (as convenient as it might be to think of them as such). Morphogenetic field enrolment is exquisitely subtle, and has much to do with individual integrity.

Psychosis

While neurosis is a relatively common experience, psychosis is a disease defined by its impact on general functionality. Psychosis may result from engagement with a pathological group essence, causing the individual to presence its essential characteristics. Psychosis is more easily recognisable, being more dramatic, but is more difficult to find a cause for, as the interaction between the mental and physical states may be obscure.

However, for the homoeopath the lack of aetiology does not present an insurmountable problem, as that is where the similimum comes into its own.

Cure in cases of psychosis is one of the most magnificent achievements of homoeopathy. Indeed, as symptomatology shifts towards the mental end of the spectrum, the likelihood of cure becomes greater. This is most clearly seen in cases of acute physical traumas, e.g. accidental injuries, which are normally attended by psychotic symptoms: screaming, crying, antisocial behaviour, moaning, etc. That is one of the reasons why acute physical trauma can be easy to prescribe to.

RESOLUTION OF KNOWN PROBLEMS

The theory of group disease naturally suggests solutions to known problems in homoeopathy, several of which are discussed below.

Resolution of epidemic diseases

Epidemic diseases have traditionally been classified as miasmatic in the classical sense. Thus, for example, HIV/AIDS would be regarded as a miasm in its own right (the human immunovirus being its vector) and a sub-type of luesis. However, you would not be able to eliminate the group disease solely by the use of the similimum, e.g. Nitricum Acidum (though the similimum might palliate admirably).

In that example, for treatment to be complete you would also need to administer the relevant group disease isopathic—Human Immunodeficiency Virus (HIV)—in potency. Thus, isotherapy is more than simply miasmatic treatment: it is the treatment of chronic disease for which the vector has been identified.

I suspect that the treatment of the patient presenting with an identifiable group disease may *always* require a multi-remedy approach, e.g. isopathy, homoeopathy, support remedies, constitutional, and so on. However, even with the best homoeopathic treatment, I am not convinced that group disease can be completely cured in the individual. It is possible that it may only be weakened to the point where it is no longer in a medical issue.

In passing, it will be observed that the resolution of all disease in the patient using only the relative miasmic has not been achieved.

Systematic development of materia medica

The development of homoeopathic materia medica is based on two kinds of provings:

- *Type A*—results of (largely) accidental toxification and infection
- *Type B*—results of experimental administrations of potentised essences.

Type A provings produce the symptoms on which many isopathic prescriptions are based, while Type B provings produce the symptoms on which homoeopathic prescriptions are made. This is a distinction the *Homoeopathic Materia Medica* has yet to make. The result is that it is not always clear from the remedy picture which symptoms, if any, might call for an isopathic.

Take, for example, mercury, whose toxicology is well established. If we look at Boericke's remedy picture of Mercurius we see that there is a wondrous mixture of toxicological and homoeopathic proving symptoms. If we consult Martindale we can discover those symptoms which were not observed during homoeopathic provings. It is these patients who may have been poisoned with mercury, and who might benefit from isopathic Mercurius and, perhaps, the nosode Mercuriosinum (though the former will prove superior).

There is a need for the *Materia Medica* to show which symptoms were not obtained by experimental proving. In the meantime, we may as well designate known sources of toxicity—Martindale, *MIMS*, *The Merck Index*, and the like—as being isopathic materia medicas. What would then be lacking, of course, would be a systematic *mental* materia medica. All group diseases *have* mental characteristics, of course; all that remains is for someone catalogue them.

A systematic programme of prophylaxis (see Part 4)

It is convenient to reconsider homoeoprophylaxis in the light of group disease theory. The chief advantage of doing so is that it establishes prophylaxis as a legitimate strategy for the treatment of *anticipation.*

The typology is of secondary relevance, and it mainly used for determining whether it should be treated homoeopathically (he is already suffering, in anticipation) or isopathically (he wishes to minimise possible future suffering), or both.

Until now, homoeopaths have not based their prophylaxis programmes on classical theory.

KEY CONCEPTS

Group disease A disease of a group. It corresponds, by a factor of scale, to an individual disease.

Group disease vector A communicable noxious influence whose establishment in the individual signals acceptance of disease.

Morphic resonance Harmonic attunement resulting in reverberative propagation, and synchronisation.

Prophylaxis homoeopathic prescribing in anticipation of a disturbance of the vital force.

Suppressive medication Medicine that is prescribed antipathically, i.e. for the purpose of preventing symptoms.

Vaccination Mass biosuppression. In allopathic medicine, the mass administration of toxic doses of biological group disease vectors, called vaccines, with the intention of suppressing symptoms.

PART 2
ISOPATHIC TECHNOLOGY

2 Isopathic pharmacognosy

3 Isopathic pharmacodynamics 1 - Modes of action

4 Isopathic pharmacodynamics 2 - Remedial dynamics

2 - ISOPATHIC PHARMACOGNOSY

THE ISOPATHIC MATERIA MEDICA
SPECIAL FEATURES OF ISOPATHIC MEDICINES
Unlimited potentisation and storage methods
Original sacrifice
Total symptom picture already known
Eliminative power expressed as potency
SOURCES OF ISOPATHIC REMEDIES
Vectors
Nosodes
FORMS OF ISOPATHIC MEDICINES
SOURCES OF PHARMACOLOGICAL DATA
INTRINSIC HEALING POTENTIAL OF REMEDIES

THE ISOPATHIC MATERIA MEDICA

The *Homoeopathic Materia Medica* is, of course, the pharmacopoeia of homoeopathics. However it is more than that, as among its contents are many common isopathics:

- the nosodes
- known disease vectors
- non-biological substances
- allopathic drugs.

The nosodes include the miasmics, and are all common group disease remedies. What the other remedies have in common is that many of them may have been made from known toxins. Normally, we do not include in the class of isopathics remedies made from harmless substances, e.g. water (even if some of them are proven homoeopathics).

The class of isopathics also includes everything that has not been subjected to proving, but which is known to be toxic (or potentially so) whether or not it is physical. The range is therefore infinite.

SPECIAL FEATURES OF ISOPATHIC MEDICINES

Isopathic medicines have the defining features of all homoeopathic medicines, as described in Book 2. In addition, they have a few notable features.

Unlimited potentisation and storage methods

Because most isopathics have been drawn from the miasmics, and have been made from nosodes, they have been manufactured and stored by traditional homoeopathic techniques. However, there is absolutely no reason why this has to be the case, given that:

- they are not usually proven (though there is no reason why they should not be subjected to proving)
- many were only potentised in the traditional way because they were originally conceived as homoeopathics

- they have been made and stored by non-standard methods (mainly radionically in the form of **analogue-icons**) for over a century (by Malcom Rae (1913-1979), and David Tansley (1934-1988)
- many are not nosodal.

Original sacrifice

Isopathics are not homoeopathic in their action on the individual, and do not require the same commemorative act of destructive potentisation as remedies intended to be proven and used homoeopathically.

But they do require essential modification, especially in the case of physical toxins, and that is normally done using potentisation. (An additional advantage of doing this is that the remedy will then have a homoeopathic action on the communicative group itself, though that is incidental and will not be discussed further.)

Total symptom picture already known

There is no need to conduct provings of isopathic remedies, as:

- their existence is based on vectors with known toxicology
- the vectors are always the vectors of the presenting group disease
- the group diseases are not mysterious, but are by definition group—societal, industrial, medical etc—phenomena
- we do not select an isopathic on the basis that it is the similimum.

Eliminative power expressed as potency

The **actual medical power** of an isopathic may be thought of as its *eliminative* power (just as that of a homoeopathic may be thought of as its *curative* power) and, like a homoeopathic, is expressed as its ***potency***. Moreover, it is calculated in the same way as the *actual curative power* of a homoeopathic medicine (see Book 1, Chapter 12).

When toxic substances are at cause, and the vital force is low, the actual eliminative potency will begin at a low number whereas when, say, a toxic *idea* is at cause a high potency may be given.

SOURCES OF ISOPATHIC REMEDIES

The sources of isopathics include:

- all known poisons
- all imaginable toxic influences, both physical and nonphysical.

In isopathy, we can consider all of the above to be vectors of disease; and we refer to remedies sourced from infected people as nosodes.

Vectors

Remedies made from harmful substances are superior to those made from infected people. The latter are made be used as isopathics, even if their traditional role is as homoeopathics, e.g. Mercurius.

Nosodes

Remedies made from infected people, tissues etc are all true isopathics, though they have traditionally been applied as though they were homoeopathic, e.g. Carcinosin: eczema in children.

FORMS OF ISOPATHIC MEDICINES

Though an intended isopathic may never have been observed before—you may be the first to use it, and there is no published isopathic materia medica as such—it is manufactured and represented pharmaceutically in the same way as a homoeopathic. The only difference is that you may not have to consult a materia medica before choosing to make one.

For example, let us say your patient presents with a candida infection. You might decide to prescribe Candida Albicans 30C together with Lycopodium 1M as a hepatoprotective.

If you don't have the candida nosode (which is made from the group disease vector) you can make it radionically. If necessary, you can even make it in the form of an autopathic (though personally I have not found it necessary to do this). You will find that all the common nosodes are available in multiple potencies from leading manufacturers.

The forms of potentised medicines are discussed more fully in Book 1.

SOURCES OF PHARMACOLOGICAL DATA

The **pharmacological data** concerning group disease remedies is drawn from:

- accidental poisonings
- homoeopathic provings
- observations of allopathic patients
- pathology reports
- reports of environmental and industrial poisonings
- toxicological and pharmacological tests of crude substances, e.g. as reported in *MIMS* and other pharmaceutical publications.

INTRINSIC HEALING POTENTIAL OF REMEDIES

In homoeopathic pharmacy we decide the appropriateness of the potency by taking into account two factors: the intrinsic curative power of the remedy (as brought to light by proving) and the vital force of the patient. In both cases we have a wealth of data to draw from.

However, in isopathic pharmacy we do not need to carry out an experimental proving of the remedy to know how noxious the source is, as its effects are often well documented. We will therefore proceed to potentise the remedy based on the patient's vital force.

The only note I would make is in regard to mentals. Often, these are not obviously the result of the effects of a vector, especially in the absence of reports from the patient. Where there is no apparent evidence of the ingestion of a vector, one would normally prescribe homoeopathically without even considering whether it is an isopathic case. But what if the homoeopathic fails? Then one must retake the case, and look for a vector.

KEY CONCEPTS

Actual medical power The product of a remedy's intrinsic curative power and its nominal numerical potency.

Analogue-icon A symbolic representation of a remedy that may be used to produce a medicine.

Pharmacological data Data obtained from toxicological and pharmacological tests of crude substances, accidental poisonings, tests on animals, homoeopathic provings, observations of hospital patients, intuitive discoveries, feedback from patients, and reports of environmental and industrial poisonings.

Potency **1.** Curative power. **2.** Magnitude of curative power expressed as a medical force indicating device (MFID), e.g. 200C.

Sarcode A remedy prepared from a healthy biological whole creature, or its tissues, secretions or excretions.

3 - ISOPATHIC PHARMACODYNAMICS 1 - MODES OF ACTION

INTRODUCTION TO ISOPATHY
The limits of isopathy
FEATURES OF THE ISOPATHIC REMEDY
Isopathic remedy as a matched morphogenetic field
Effect on higher-level morphogenetic field
Basis for selection
Isopathic not to be used when the similimum is required
Isopathic may double as similimum
Function
Clinical features
MODAL DYNAMICS
ELIMINATIVE MODE
Eliminative function of the isopathic
Single prescribing criterion
Apparent aggravation
Mistaking the isopathic for the similimum
Prophylaxis in the elimination mode

INTRODUCTION TO ISOPATHY

Isopathy is the use of potentialised medicines on the principle that a specific and not generic (i.e. similar) remedial match will result in the annihilation of a form of resistance that is identifiable with a *group disease*.

As every group disease is identifiable by its vector, isopathics are often prescribed for the specific purpose of eliminating the vectors themselves—in detoxification, for example—as if they were the *cause* of disease.

The limits of isopathy

Despite its tremendous utility, isopathy has limitations as a therapy (as does homoeopathy). In particular:

- it is not curative
- it will not completely clear a case of toxicity from—or predisposition to—a given species of disease
- unless either the aetiology or vector is known, it will not work
- its effects and prescriptive rationale do not conform to homoeopathic theorems.

FEATURES OF THE ISOPATHIC REMEDY

Isopathic remedy as a matched morphogenetic field

The ***group disease remedy*** is—as are all remedies—simply a matched morphogenetic field, differing from a homoeopathic remedy only in the exactitude of its selection.

Whereas a homoeopathic medicine is made from a potentised remedy that matches (is the similimum for) the patient's symptom picture, an isopathic medicine is made from the potentised disease vector itself or, if it may not be easily isolated, from an individual who has the disease, in the form of a nosode (referred to as an ***autopathic*** when that individual is the patient himself).

It is therefore the therapy of choice for a group disease, as it matches (is the 'similimum' for) the symptom picture for the *entire group*.

Effect on higher-level morphogenetic field

It is important to note that an isopathic qua isopathic, is designed not to *cure* the presenting disease, but to weaken the related higher-level morphogenetic field influence.

Thus, the remedy *for the susceptible group* is actually prescribed to the individual patient *isopathically* as the solution to his presentation (without being similimum). Thus, *the isopathic is to the* ***group disease*** *as the similimum is to the individual disease.*

Theoretically, the group disease would eventually lose its force if the curative effect became strong enough. This effect—so-called herd immunity—is not the result of resistance, but is due to conductivity (or health).

Basis for selection

An isopathic medicine is a potency that has been selected for its original isomorphism to the presenting pathophysiology. For example, in a case of malaria the potency might be made from malarial infection, i.e. a nosode.

To the homoeopath, two things will be immediately apparent: first, the isopathic is not selected for its resemblance to the total symptom picture, and second (which follows from the first) it is not the similimum. It further follows that it cannot bring about cure.

Thus, the term *group disease isopathic* refers to a remedy that is routinely prescribed for patients who share a recognised specific group disease *vector*. All other remedies are regarded as either similimums or constitutionals.

Isopathy not to be used when similimum required

Isopathy is only indicated when the presentation indicates an **obstacle to cure** that *must* be dealt with before homoeopathic treatment can proceed. Evidence of an underlying delusional or pathophysiological state is not a barrier to immediate homoeopathic treatment. If a patient comes to you with a symptom picture which perfectly matches a given homoeopathic remedy, then that is what he must have.

All patients have underlying delusional or pathophysiological states: that is human life for you. Your job is to cure what may be cured, if that is what the patient wants.

Isopathic may double as similimum

Of course, if a group disease **isopathic** has *proven symptoms*, it may double as a similimum, e.g. Tuberculinum Bovinum. It almost goes without saying that, where such a *bi-modal* remedy is indicated it is probable that the underlying disease influence is familial. Also, in such cases any failure of the nosode to complete the case would invariably call for a related homoeopathic.

Function

So far we have said nothing about disease as a vital disturbance, and that is because the connection of isopathy to disease is tenuous, and lies in its function. If the function of an isopathic is not to cure the individual patient, then what is it? It is to weaken the patient's connection to the relevant pathological morphogenetic field (a connection that constitutes an obstacle to cure).

This, in turn, will have the effect of eliminating the relevant disease vector, ameliorating the patient, and preparing the vital force for homoeotherapy. It is therefore a first line therapy for chronic disease.

Clinical features

Being a medicine, the isopathic displays pharmocodynamic features. However, despite being made from a potentised essence, it is often not made from a proven remedy. Thus, we might not find it in the homoeopathic materia medica. Nor do we need to prove it in order to educe its eliminative medical power, as that is indicated by its source. However, like a homoeopathic, it does display certain clinical features:

- *modality*—the ability of all remedies to display modal dynamics, e.g. elimination
- *functionality*—the ability of all remedies to perform a variety of clinical functions, e.g. isotherapy
- *specificity*—invariable conformity to type and species, i.e. pharmacognostic reliability in accordance with accepted toxicological data
- *exquisiteness*—criticality of pharmacy, e.g. the prescriptive rigour that is required to ensure the desired posological result.

We will discuss now look at the first of these: **modality**.

MODAL DYNAMICS

In Book 1(Chapter 9), it was explained that potentised remedies display eight modes of action: susceptive, amplificational, curative, palliative, eliminative, supportive, restorative, and probative (see *Key Concepts*, below). Only two of these, the curative and restorative modes, may result in a curative restoration of the vital force, while another, the probative mode, is designed to find out what a remedy may cure.

The remaining modes may all be seen in isopathy, but only one —the **eliminative mode**—routinely results in the elimination of group disease vectors. It is therefore in this mode that isopathics have their principle action.

The rest of this chapter will be devoted to discussing this mode of action, while the next chapter will deal with other features of isopathics.

ELIMINATIVE MODE

The group disease has a distinct form that, according to the vitalistic hypothesis, evokes from nature (the externality to which it aspires) a distinct remedy called a *group disease isopathic*. Once it has installed itself in an individual organism, a group disease may be to some extent dispelled by that isopathic. Every dispelling on an individual scale will also have the effect of weakening the communicability of the disease generally in the endemic group.

Eliminative function of the isopathic

Whereas a remedy that is prescribed homoeopathically has the function of cure, one that is prescribed isopathically has the function of empowering the organism to conduct a specific influence. Its special value is therefore in assisting the organism to either generate or eliminate a particular *unwanted* influence.

Should the organism then become symptom free, it does not necessarily mean that the group disease remedy acted homoeopathically, but rather in the role of pseudo-chronic disease eliminator. Of course, in the presence of continued exposure to the causative factor, that disease would reoccur.

Single prescribing criterion

It must be remembered that a potentised remedy is not isopathic per se, but only to the extent that it is *prescribed* isopathically. Thus, a prescription of Arsenicum Album in a case of arsenic toxicity would have the effect of acting isopathically and causing the elimination of, say, industrially ingested arsenic.

However, it does not follow that it would be correct, in that example, to prescribe that remedy homoeopathically. For homoeopathic prescribing the similimum needs to be sought, and it will always be found to correspond to the total symptom picture.

Apparent aggravation

Medicating a patient isopathically for the purpose of stimulating the elimination of a particular substance will usually cause the organism to release that substance into the most convenient channel of elimination. This could result in unexpected symptoms, frequently a temporary increase in or return of toxicosis—actually, an isopathic aggravation—which may necessitate palliative homoeopathic treatment. In the meantime, vectors would continue to be eliminated.

Conduction, i.e. elimination, also occurs in response to homoeotherapy, of course, though it is virtually impossible to predict the metabolic results, due to their complexity. In using isotherapy, on the other hand, one is primarily interested in the effect of the isopathic on a substance that has *already* been identified, so that the physiological result is often predictable.

Unwanted *non-curative* aggravation due to the elimination of the original noxious influence into the bloodstream should always be anticipated, and may even point to a contraindication for the use of a particular isopathic, depending on the nature of the toxic influence.

Note that *new* symptoms often point to a proving, which may be amenable to palliation.

(This topic is further discussed under *Isopathic provings*, in the next chapter, and *Direct and indirect elimination*, in Chapter 6.)

Mistaking the isopathic for the similimum

When the patient presents with a group disease which has an identifiable vector that seems also to be the homoeopathic similimum, that remedy will act primarily as an isopathic and *not* as a homoeopathic. In effect, it will have been chosen on the basis of faulty rationale.

Example Set 3.1 Mistaking the group disease isopathic for the similimum

Ex.	*Scenario*	*Group disease isopathic*	*Example of similimum*
1	Wilson's disease	Cuprum Metallicum	Nux Vomica
2	Cigarette addiction	Nicotinum	Absinthium
3	Cardiac arrhythmia	Coffea	Chamomilla
4	Cancer	Carcinosinum	Arsenicum

The fault lies not with the prescriber, but may be attributed to the *Homoeopathic Materia Medica* and the Homoeopathic Repertory, for failing to make this distinction. This has, I believe, been the cause of a great deal of failure in homoeotherapy, because an isopathic is not implicitly curative for the individual (and many homoeopathics may be used as isopathics, especially the nosodes).

In Example Set 3.1 we see this error hard at work in four case scenarios.

Scenario 1: Wilson's disease

In the first case, the patient has presented with Wilson's disease, a genetic disorder that results in the accumulation of copper in the body. The similimum may seem to be Cuprum Metallicum, however this is a disease with a known vector, i.e. copper.

When administered as the primary remedy it will therefore act as an isopathic, causing a lowering of toxic copper levels (which may be the best that the patient could ever hope for). The role of the homoeopathic may not become apparent until the patient begins to improve, when other symptoms may emerge.

On the other hand, if we ignore the group disease scenario and prescribe Cuprum Metallicum as a similimum we will still see the elimination effect, and possibly a degree of amelioration, but may never achieve cure. This may lead us to conclude either that the remedy was incorrect, or that the potency was insufficient. The first conclusion might be more fruitful if it results in a reconsideration of the case. For example, perhaps the similimum for the individual might turn out to be Nux Vomica. (But note that this is a case of genetic disorder, which may not be amenable to curative therapy.)

Scenario 2: Cigarette addiction

The patient has presented with cardiac arrhythmia. The similimum seems to be Nicotinum, which makes sense to the practitioner, as the patient is addicted to cigarettes. However, in view of the cigarette addiction admitted by the patient, it can't be regarded as the correct remedy for that patient. That is because it is actually the similimum for the *group* disease.

In this case, Nicotinum causes a sudden elimination of cigarette toxins into the bloodstream, causing a history of seizure disorder to reappear. After retaking the case, the true similimum is arrived at, say, Absinthium.

Scenario 3: Cardiac arrhythmia

The patient has presented with a coffee addiction, resulting in undesirable side effects. The homoeopath has no hesitation in prescribing Coffea, which only aggravates severely. The solution turns out to be Chamomilla.

Scenario 4: Cancer

The patient has been diagnosed with cancer, and comes from a history of familial cancer. The similimum seems to be Carcinosinum, which produces contradictory and alternating symptom pictures, but no amelioration, despite high potencies. Only a more carefully prescribed remedy, perhaps Arsenicum, will work.

In this case, the first remedy had indeed been working, but as an *isopathic* which, with this particular remedy, can have unexpected side effects while it is dispelling the group influence.

Of course, as with all group disease prescriptions, it is only possible to see if the remedy has cleared the pathophysiology if the patient *no longer has it*. And then there will invariably be the aftermath to consider, e.g. allopathically generated problems. In this case, the homoeopathic alone will ameliorate, but with the group disease itself still in place, there may be a return of cancer symptoms, especially if there has been artificial suppression.

Notes on the above cases

1. In each case there would be less of a problem if the presentation had been assessed as a group disease in the first place, which may or may not require isopathy, but which would at least facilitate the creation of a treatment strategy.
2. Though there is benefit in each case from the similimum it is not curative but palliative.
3. The complete solution would be to prescribe the isopathic with at least one support homoeopathic (possibly the remedies indicated in the examples).
4. Naturopathic solutions are probably indicated.

Prophylaxis in the elimination mode

At the beginning of prophylactic therapy the patient may experience a slight amplification of the vital force followed by some elimination, though it should be barely noticeable after the healing gradient (a posological concept introduced in Book 1) has been established. The experience is due to the elimination of *anticipation* of illness (which is simply the patient's morphogenic field resonating with that of the disease).

KEY CONCEPTS

Autopathic A potentialised medicine made from the patient himself.

Eliminative mode Mode of medicinal action in which the patient exhibits increased mental and emotional activity, with physiological elimination. The primary mode of isopathy.

Group disease A disease of a group. It corresponds, by a factor of scale, to an individual disease.

Group disease remedy A signature remedy which is evoked by the diseased group from nature (the externality to which it aspires), and which belongs to the family of isopathics.

Healing gradient **1.** The natural inclination of the organism to heal. **2.** The inclination to heal that is automatically installed when a potentialised medicine is administered.

Isopathic Of a medicine, being made from the same species that which caused the disease.

Isopathy Treatment of group disease by administering a potentised group disease vector.

Modality **1.** An ameliorating or aggravating factor. **2.** A therapeutic approach. **3.** A remedial display of modal dynamics, e.g. cure.

Modes of medicinal response There are eight: amplificational, curative, eliminative, palliative, probative, restorative, supportive, and susceptive (see each, separately).

Obstacle to cure Any factor that impedes cure.

4 - ISOPATHIC PHARMACODYNAMICS 2 - REMEDIAL DYNAMICS

MINOR MODAL CHANGES
Susceptive mode
Curative mode
Amplificational mode
CENTRALITY OF DISTURBANCE
CLINICAL FEATURES OF ISOPATHIC MEDICINES
MEDICINAL FUNCTIONALITY AND APPLICATIONS
Group disease treatment
Allergy and hypersensitivity reactions
Euthenic therapy
Vaccinosis
Aftermath of group disease
Detoxification
Prophylaxis
SPECIFICITY
Morphic equality
PHARMACEUTICAL CRITICALITY
Isopathic provings
Enhancement of intrinsic non-curative action
Healing gradient
Negative gradient
The single remedy
Polypharmacy

Minimum potency

Demands of the social dimension

Vitoequivalence factor

Single dose

Initiating dose

Maintenance doses

REPEATABILITY

REMEDY SIGNATURE

AUTOPATHY

CONSTITUTIONAL ISOTHERAPY

The constitutional doubling as an isopathic

Elimination of diathetic features

MINOR MODAL CHANGES

At any time during isopathic therapy—and remember that elimination is normally undertaken *prior to* homoeopathic treatment—a change of modality may be indicated by the symptom picture.

Susceptive mode

I have found that the susceptive mode can take much longer to complete when using isopathics, not so much in detoxification cases, but in cases of communicable diseases and other forms of infection. In these cases the starting potency might have to be higher than one would expect to use. Still, it is always necessary to install the healing gradient in order to enable elimination. Once that has been initiated, of course, the remedy will be seen to work in the eliminative mode.

Curative mode

When detoxification or group disease (classical: *miasmic*) therapy has begun, a change in the total symptom picture will occur. Typically, one observes:

- new symptoms
- a clearer definition of the symptom picture
- an increase in the vital force.

When that happens, the similimum must be sought. Note that the correct remedy will no longer be the indicated isopathic.

Amplificational mode

When the symptom picture is too vague to prescribe on, the constitutional remedy—providing it is known—may be given in low potency. It will act in the amplificational mode to cause an increase in the vital force and with it the total symptom picture. The isopathic may then be given with confidence if it is indicated.

CENTRALITY OF DISTURBANCE

As we saw in Chapter 1, the centre of disturbance of a group disease cannot be within the patient's morphogenetic field, otherwise it would be susceptible to neutralisation by the similimum, and that is not the case. It must therefore be within a higher-level morphogenetic field, one of a social nature (but having no location, despite having possible local associations).

Thus, we can assume that, if an isopathic has any *curative* effect, it is somehow within the higher-level field. Holistic theory actually provides for interpenetrating fields, which allows us to see how pathogenic morphic fields enrol susceptible lower-level fields. In the case of disease the lower-level field subscribes to the disease field, then allows itself to receive disease vectors, which are the clinical 'brand' of the particular infection or contamination.

The isopathic that is indicated for the individual does not neutralise the higher-level field—else that group disease would cease to exist—but it does weaken the morphic bond. We might speculate that this is the point at which individual cure takes place.

CLINICAL FEATURES OF ISOPATHIC MEDICINES

In the preceding chapter, we listed the clinical features of isopathic medicines, and discussed the first and most important of these: modality. The following clinical features have relevance to isopathy, and will be discussed below:

- *functionality*—the ability to perform a variety of clinical functions
- *specificity*—invariable conformity to type and species, i.e. pharmacognostic reliability in accordance with accepted toxicological data
- *exquisiteness*—criticality of pharmacy, e.g. the prescriptive rigour that is required to ensure the desired posological result.

MEDICINAL FUNCTIONALITY AND APPLICATIONS

An isopathic has only one function: to weaken the resonance which the patient's morphogenetic field has with the enrolling morphogenetic field (which may be thought of as a group disease field). In doing so it eliminates the group disease vector, or agent, from the patient and paves the way for homoeopathic treatment. Three clinical applications of that function will be discussed:

- group disease treatment
- detoxification
- prophylaxis.

Group disease treatment

The elimination of the influences of group disease could be said to be the main aim of isotherapy. The isopathic approach to group disease is to eliminate from the organism specific morphogenetic fields: those associated with identifiable group disease vectors. Often, this step will follow naturopathic detoxification. Any remaining toxic influences may be removed by the prescription of the signature isopathic remedy in potency.

Allergy and hypersensitivity reactions

Allergy is evidence that the body is unable to harmlessly conduct a substance or influence. Illness is impossible when conduction is perfect, and certain when its opposite, resistance, is present. In allergy, the allergen may encounter total resistance, in which case the patient may die if left untreated.

It has been held by physiologists that the immune system is mechanism for resisting disease. In fact, a perfectly healthy adult would be a superconductor, and incapable of becoming ill except by physical injury. The correct attunement of the human organism to itself and its environment would result in a state of zero allergic potential. Homoeotherapy does not increase resistance: it removes it.

In **hyposensitisation** homoeopathics, especially in combination with isopathics, are used to desensitise patients to a wide range of substances, from environmental substances, e.g. air pollution, to phobia objects, e.g. birds.

(For potency selection in hyposensitisation, see Chapter 8.)

Euthenic therapy

In obstetric homoeopathy, **euthenic therapy** is the use of potentialised medicines to eliminate group disease influences from a female patient in preparation for or during pregnancy.

The traditional form of euthenic therapy is a series of antimiasmatic treatments during the first trimester of pregnancy aimed at the elimination of the classic miasms. However, euthenic therapy may be used to eliminate any unwanted influence during or in anticipation of pregnancy. An example programme is at Example Set 4.1.

Note that euthenic therapy should not be used as a substitute for simple detoxification, which might be inappropriate during pregnancy, depending on the anticipated results. Neither should it be used as a kind of simulated homoeoprophylaxis.

The ideal remedies to use would be nosodes. Some authors have suggested the use, instead or in addition, of miasmic homoeopathics, e.g. Sulphur for the psoric miasm, Natrum Sulphuricum for the sycotic miasm, etc. However, that is not the purpose of these remedies, and may simply produce a proving, with one possible exception, namely when the remedy under consideration is the constitutional.

In that case, the remedy, if given, could have the effect of bringing to light a diathetic symptom picture, which could then be confidently prescribed to. The net effect would be the removal of underlying or potential pathology.

Example Set 4.1 Euthenic programme

Week	*Scenario*	*Therapeutic strategy*
1	Family history of tuberculosis	Tuberculinum Bovinum
2	Individual history of recurrent influenza	Influenzinum
3	Family history of cancer	Carcinosinum

Notes:

1. The programme is worked out in consultation with the patient.
2. The constitutional may be given at any time during the programme, but only once, in high potency.
3. The traditional (miasmic) therapeutic model calls for a different miasmic nosode each week for four weeks with or without other remedies.

(For potency selection in euthenic therapy, see Chapter 8.)

Vaccinosis

Isotherapy may be preferred to homoeotherapy as the first-line treatment for **vaccinosis**, as it will promote the elimination of the relevant group disease vector, whereas a homoeopathic, e.g. Thuja Occidentalis, would not (though there might be minor elimination, including the vector itself). Nevertheless, homoeotherapy will be inevitable at some point. (See also *Vaccinosis*, in Chapter 7.)

Aftermath of group disease

An isopathic may also be indicated by the presencing by the patient of the *aftermath* of a group disease, e.g. a Medorrhinum presentation with a history of gonorrhoea which had been treated allopathically. The action of the isopathic would be to cause elimination of the group disease influence. Thus, the sheer predictability of isopathy greatly supports its use.

Detoxification

All potentialised medicines cause elimination, which is defined as the release of toxins accompanying the annihilation of resistance. The toxins will be those which it is within the power of the organism to remove (given the homoeopathic used), where a toxin is defined as anything physical or non-physical that naturally causes the vital force to become either distorted or stalled, and which remains present in the patient. Thus, in the course of healing detoxification will occur naturally, usually in a number of ways.

This effect can be exploited, especially isopathically, to remove specific toxins, noxious influences, etc, and to increase the eliminating power of specific organs. (This is the principle behind miasmatic therapy.)

In general, even in the absence of isotherapy, incidental homoeopathic detoxification will occur and, providing a good history has been taken, may be anticipated. Incidental homoeopathic detoxification may require careful anticipation where it is suspected that harmful substances, e.g. psychotropic drugs, may have been stored by the body, as these may be released into the bloodstream during detoxification.

Isopathic detoxification has been mentioned in various parts of this series, in particular:

In Book 2:
Chapter 8: *Practical potency selection*
Chapter 12: *Obstacles to cure*
Chapter 10: *Review and second prescription*

In this book:
Chapter 1: *Group disease (*see *Environmental disorders)*
Chapter 6: *Isopathic detoxification*
Chapter 7: *Iatrogenic disorders.*

Prophylaxis
For the prophylactic applications of isopathics, see Chapters 9-10.

SPECIFICITY

Remedy specificity is invariable conformity to type and species, i.e. pharmacognostic reliability in accordance with accepted toxicological data. Unlike a homoeopathic, an isopathic will not bring cure, given a specific remedy and case totality. What it *will* elicit is a specific elimination response, based on what is known about the patient's pathophysiology and the nature of the toxicity. The prescription is made on the basis of morphic equality, not morphic similarity.

Morphic equality
A remedy selected on the basis of essential *sameness* will act primarily in the eliminative mode to reduce the influence of a given noxious morphogenetic field, and also its signature group disease vector (and group disease vectors of sufficient similarity).

For example, Thallium Metallicum will eliminate the unwanted thallium morphic field (and with it, thallium) from the individual. However, that would only be the beginning of therapy, as homoeotherapy would also be in order, and selection of the correct remedy would then depend on the total symptom picture.

We would also see the same kind of result with any of the human nosodes in potency. They all act isopathically, which is the basis for miasm therapy.

Several points need to be made:

- Any isopathic, being a potentialised medicine, can produce an accidental proving. If no experimental proving has been recorded, the symptoms may be unfamiliar, especially the mentals. Antidoting would be done *homoeopathically*, and should present no difficulties.
- An isopathic will not remove a group disease (classical: *miasm*) the way a homoeopathic removes a disease, i.e. by pranic neutralisation. Instead, it will weaken the morphic resonance of the entraining morphic field. It is able to do this because it is *itself* a resonant morphic field, one which has been selected for its exact resonance.
- In the case of an **autopathic** (see below), the necessary condition of identicality of the autopathic is not required.

PHARMACEUTICAL CRITICALITY

Whereas every potentised remedy that has been created for homoeopathic use has clearly demonstrated its pharmaceutical exquisiteness through the proving process, and its clinical application through its clinical use, the same cannot be said of every remedy used in the isopathic mode, hence the following comments.

Isopathic provings

The pharmaceutical criticality of isopathics, i.e. the morphic relationship of the specific features of the *source* of the potency—especially its toxicity—to the specific features of the patient for whom it might be suitable, have not been tested. However, note the following:

- Some classic isopathics *have* been subject to experimental provings in potency, and have been included in the homoeopathic materia medica. The main advantage of this is that we know their modalities, and often their mentals, making clinical provings relatively easy to spot.
- Non-homoeopathic toxicological records—these are actually provings of non-potentised substances—have always existed, and may be found within seconds on the internet, usually without mentals.
- All of the actions of allopathic drugs, whether designed or unintended, i.e. through side effects, are provings.
- All of the actions of recreational drugs are provings.
- The patient's presentation is itself evidence of a proving.

Enhancement of intrinsic non-curative action

Toxins my be straightforward in their effects (e.g. many chemical poisons), or they may be insidious, e.g. many noxious morphogenetic fields, especially those having biological vectors. But they each have a certain vitality, ranging from the distinct, e.g snake venom, to the indistinct, e.g. political abuse.

Usually, that vitality is so well known that experimental proving is unnecessary. Potentising in order to enhance the essence's intrinsic non-curative action is therefore straightforward.

(The reader may with to review Book 2, Chapter 10, which introduces these concepts.)

Healing gradient

What we are looking for is a sign that the healing gradient has been successfully installed, and that is achieved by a potency just high enough, given the patient's vital force, and a dosage sufficient to provide it.

With an isopathic, we always know that the remedy was correctly selected, so the only considerations are potency and dosage.

Negative gradient

Note that both positive and negative pranic gradients may be created by medication. Iatrogenic disease, for example, is created by the installation of a *positive* gradient, i.e. one that has the effect of *increasing* resistance to the natural flow of prana.

The single remedy

In contrast to homoeopathy, there is no rule in isopathy that only one remedy be prescribed (though it should be unnecessary, in any case). (See *Polypharmacy*, below.)

Polypharmacy

In isotherapy it is permissible to use polypharmacy in the following circumstances:

- *detoxification (1)*—an isopathic as the primary, and a homoeopathic as a secondary, should the need arise, i.e. as an organ support remedy
- *detoxification (2)*—a primary isopathic plus a homoeopathic for symptoms of sickness due to the toxin being eliminated
- *detoxification (3)*—multiple toxicities, say, from an industrial setting, requiring multiple isopathic remedies
- *prophylaxis (1)*—a complex of prophylactics, say, for an intended traveller
- *prophylaxis (2)*—a complex of prophylactics—the circumstances are various— accompanied by homoeopathic stand-by remedies
  prophylaxis (3)—an antenatal complex
- *euthenics*—standard euthenic prescribing, usually as a complex, to remove inherited group disease (classical: *miasm*)
- *miasmic elimination, with or without a protective homoeopathic*
- *acute group disease, e.g. the effects of a new epidemic infection.* (Often the homoeopath reaches for an old standby, but overlooks the need to eliminate the known group disease vector using a nosode while he has the opportunity.)
- *iatrogenic disease treatment.*

Minimum potency

Demands of the social dimension

The social dimension of a group disease means that, except when acute in nature it will be both powerful and insidious. It will therefore demand some respect, and that, in turn will necessitate low initial potencies (with the possible exception of diseases of a psychiatric nature).

Even so, one has to be carefully not to attempt explosive elimination in cases where the symptom picture displays, for example, anger. (I have included this caveat for practitioners who may be unused to isopathy, and who might be accustomed to seeing powerful emotions neutralised harmlessly by such remedies as Chamomilla.)

Vitoequivalence factor

In Book 2 (Chapter 10) the importance of matching the proposed homoeopathic to the patient's vital force was discussed. Each remedy has its own intrinsic vitality, which may be gauged from the *Materia Medica* entry. However, most isopathics have not been proven, so my advice is to simply match the potency to the patient's vital force.

Single dose

As far as dosage goes, the single dose rule of homoeopathy does not apply—the experimental work simply has not been done. However, because the isopathic is a remedy in potency, it will have an effect on the central disturbance.

Initiating dose

An isopathic will work in any potency. However it will still benefit from the installation of a healing gradient, just not optimally.

Maintenance doses

Amelioration will hopefully take the form of a lessening of the symptoms of the group disease. Complete disappearance will not be accomplished without some kind of homoeopathic (and often naturopathic) support.

Maintenance of the healing gradient may be done with a *collective ascending dose*, using *plussing*. If the patient's symptoms worsen, that is an aggravation. If new symptoms appear, that would normally signal a proving of the remedy.

REPEATABILITY

The action of a homoeopathic in any given case is independent of the circumstances of the case, i.e. the constitutional, the symptom picture, the internal pathophysiology etc. The action is purely one of neutralisation of the central disturbance, and this is an effect that is predictable. We could say that the similimum includes in its nature the patient's disease typology.

This is not the case with the isopathic: it does not include in its nature, or reference, the patient's individualising typology; its nature is the nature of the group disease. Once we give the remedy, we do not know exactly what will happen. That is because the patient may, and probably will, have underlying disturbances, which will come to light as the effect of the group disease subsides. Then we must consider homoeopathic solutions.

REMEDY SIGNATURE

It is the source of the remedy that has the signature, not the isopathic remedy itself. And we can therefore tell by examining the patient what the signature of his group disease looks like. Naturally, if the remedy we select has been homoeopathically proved, we will have even more information about the signature of the source, but not the remedy to be given, which is essentially *the same*. As always, the focus in isopathy is not on identifying the remedy as such but on diagnosing the group disease.

AUTOPATHY

The only true autopathic is an isopathic manufactured by using the patient himself as the base substance. (This has been called by some an 'autoisopathic', but that is an unnecessary distinction.) Traditionally, autopathics are made from eliminated substances, e.g. sputum, pus, blood or urine. In that they are invariably potencies of a diseased organism, they are nosodes.

An autopathic does not need to be made from a physical substance. It could, for example, be manufactured from a proxy, e.g. the patient's photograph. (Successes have been reported using this system, but invariably the similimum had already been administered.)

In passing, it should be noted that an autopathic is not a 'tautopathic', which is a popular misnomer for a potentised allopathic drug. Such a remedy might end up being used as both a homoeopathic and an isopathic medicine. Provings abound.

(For a discussion of potency selection, see Chapter 8.)

CONSTITUTIONAL ISOTHERAPY

The constitutional doubling as an isopathic

Amplification of the vital force following administration of the constitutional and before the completion of therapy is a normal response, and indicates the existence of blockage of the vital force which may require further treatment. Indeed, this is the main use of a constitutional.

The reason the constitutional can have a dramatic effect is because it may be *isopathic* to the constitutional diathesis (and therefore, homoeopathic to the diathetic *group*, e.g. the scrofulous type).

With that in mind, the constitutional may be prescribed for isopathic purposes in circumstances where there is a history of *known or suspected* constitution-related disease which the practitioner believes might be relieved by the similimum, if only that disease could be brought to light.

For example, a patient might present with frequent recurrent asthma and a familial history of tuberculosis. The patient's asthma is relieved by Kalium Nitricum (which is the similimum), but only temporarily. However, the putative constitutional is Tuberculinum which, when given, produces an *amplified elimination* in the form of a new symptom picture, which responds to a new similimum: Ferrum Phosphoricum. With only occasional maintenance doses of the constitutional, and perhaps occasional treatment with the new similimum, the recurrences become rare.

Note a) that the constitution may only be used as an isopathic when it is the appropriate *group disease* (classical: *miasm*) remedy, and b) that it will still tend to amplify as well as eliminate.

Elimination of diathetic features

It would be pointless to prescribe the constitutional isopathically in order to eliminate an unwanted constitutional feature, e.g. a tendency to asthma, as that is something the patient is stuck with. That said, the constitutional would tend to amplify any residual constitution-related disease, e.g. allopathically suppressed asthmatic symptoms, allowing homoeopathic treatment to take place. The constitutional feature would remain.

KEY CONCEPTS

Autopathic A potentialised medicine made from the patient himself.

Euthenic therapy In obstetric homoeopathy, the use of potentialised medicines to remove group disease influence from the mother.

Healing gradient **1.** The natural inclination of the organism to heal. **2.** The inclination to heal that is automatically installed when a potentialised medicine is administered.

Hyposensitisation Isopathic treatment designed to desensitise patients to substances.

Specific A remedy (usually one of several) that is indicated by a clinical diagnosis.

Vaccinosis The generic group disease caused by vaccination.

PART 3
SOLUTIONS TO GROUP DISEASE

5 Group disease treatment
6 Isopathic detoxification
7 Iatrogenic disorders
8 Isopathic potency selection

5 - GROUP DISEASE TREATMENT

INTRODUCTION
CHOICE OF STRATEGY
Order of prescribing
PHARMACEUTICAL OPTIONS
Case study
Strategic considerations
Autopathic solution
HEALING PATTERNS
Primary detoxification
Steady cure scenario
Underlying group disease scenario
The general result
Residual group disease influence
Homoeoprophylaxis
CASE REVIEW
POSSIBLE PRESCRIBING OUTCOMES
Amelioration
Aggravation followed by amelioration
Amelioration followed by relapse
Isopathic aggravation
Prolonged aggravation
No change
Accidental proving
New symptoms
ANTIDOTING

INTRODUCTION

This chapter, which deals with the therapeutic approach to group disease, requires of the reader that he entertain a new set of medical concepts concerning diagnosis and prescribing.

The motivating principal behind group disease therapy will be familiar to the reader via miasm theory: the desirability of ridding the organism of noxious influences. However, group disease theory redefines disease itself as possessing an additional, morphogenetic dimension.

Moreover, group disease theory is not limited to conditions that are acquired by infection, genetic inheritance and in utero events; in fact, it is not limited at all. And in that sense, it is a general theory of disease. Thus, its formulation required no revision of homoeopathic philosophy, and in fact offers an expansion of therapeutic possibility.

Paradoxically, that expansion requires of the homoeopathic physician that he consider the possibility of toxicity as an allopath might. If he is to rid the organism of what is admittedly an obstacle to cure, then he must have some knowledge, no matter now crude, of that toxic influence.

Naturally, should he decide to proceed along purely homoeopathic lines, i.e. without applying isopathic principles, he must succeed until he comes up against the obstacle to cure that the group disease presents. This difficulty will, of course, always be mitigated by the use of homoeopathics that are naturally associated with that group disease.

CHOICE OF STRATEGY

In practice, all of the following solutions may be found useful in any given case of group disease:

- several homoeopathics
- at least one isopathic
- just one autopathic.

Of these, the homoeopathics (which will be found to be in family relationship to the isopathic) will palliate or cure, and will weaken the relationship of the patient to the group. However, they will not weaken the susceptibility to the disease itself, as that is constitutional; it could therefore reoccur.

The isopathic, on the other hand, will at least partially dissolve the relationship of the patient with the group by eradicating the exogenous toxin that defines the disease's communicability.

Note that the use of the family of autopathics unique to the individual: blood, skin, saliva, etc, may, when well chosen, endow the individual physical body with additional vitality, but they will not annihilate the group disease bond, which always resists the individual's free expression.

It is not necessary to medicate all of the members of a group in order to give them all healing. Each individual act of medication has a significant effect in the group, owing to its power to exponentially influence other members. A group is not simply a number of individuals, after all, but an organic relationship. As such it is another manifestation of the life force.

Consider that when we medicate the individual patient with a homoeopathic medicine, the method by which it is dispensed is relatively unimportant. Every vitalistic medicine acts on the life force as a whole (hence the term holistic).

Order of prescribing

Given that the aim of medical treatment is to relieve suffering, the preferred homoeopathic strategy is one that addresses the most troublesome symptoms. These will be the ones that tax the patient's healing powers the hardest, so he will be better off without them. It is for this reason that obstacles to the cure of *the condition displaying the most troublesome symptoms* are removed first.

The treatment of group disease requires first that one remember the order of treatment:

- removal of obstacles to cure (plus palliative support)
- removal of toxins that will prevent cure (plus palliative support)
- addressing the central disturbance.

Some examples follow.

Scenario 1

A pulmonary (classical: *tubercular*) patient presents with erysipelas indicative of Silica. On the face of it, there would be no need to prescribe a miasmatic, say, Tuberculinum when Silica would do.

However, it might be argued that any remedy that is capable of causing an amplified radiation of symptoms must be a more centralised, and therefore, apt remedy. However, apart from the special use of the constitutional, or of a group disease isopathic to render vague symptoms more visible—in other words, to produce an artificially acute symptom picture where there had been none to speak of—we would not lead with a remedy that was not designed to produce cure.

Scenario 2

A miner presents with adhesive capsulitis complicated by apparently unrelated industrial lead toxicity. He is treated on the basis of the acute presentation with, say, Rhus Toxicodendron 200C.

Naturally, were the same patient to present primarily with, say, colitis, the treatment strategy would probably require extra consideration, as spontaneous detoxification could be expected to follow amelioration of the acute presentation, causing new acute symptoms of toxicity to appear.

Scenario 3

The patient's group disease is not readily identifiable with a common pathogen or toxin. The presentation might range from something reminiscent of a genus of disease, e.g. influenza, to a confusion of symptoms that demand analysis, or at least clarification. Often, this is the only type of presentation the patient has, in spite of successful homoeopathic prescribing over a long period of time. In such patients it often becomes apparent that the remedies prescribed have certain common dimensions that suggest a known group disease.

In this case, detoxification is not, on the face of it, indicated, nor is a group disease isopathic, because of the lack of specificity. We might, if the symptoms are weak and ill-defined, and the evidence for a specific group disease strong, use the constitutional to amplify the picture.

PHARMACEUTICAL OPTIONS

There are two types of isopathic remedies: the group disease vector and the nosode. While the potentised group disease vector might not eliminate the particular group disease completely, it will cause the organism to eliminate the vector, if it is present.

The vector itself does not bind; rather, it is its *acceptance* that bonds. Thus, elimination of the vector, while improving the patient's health, may not remove the disease. However, it might succeed to the degree that the problem disappears.

The nosode, on the other hand, will cause the expression of the group disease influence, which is usually visual in form of symptomatology. That can only be accomplished by prescribing the nosode, though note that it may not eliminate the vector.

It will now be apparent in what way group prescribing supersedes miasmic prescribing. It relieves the homoeopath of the burden of deciding which miasm or combination of miasms to prescribe, or of deciding between a nosode (made from say, pus) and a potentised vector (made from, say, the original microorganism). Group disease strategy would allow him to prescribe the vector or its pathological product, or both.

Thus, because group disease remedies, i.e. isopathics, do not require proving, we have, in respect of every group disease, the option of prescribing the vector in potency, or the nosode, providing of course that it may be obtained.

Case study

Chronic bronchitis in a smoker.

Strategic considerations

The homoeopath might identify the similimum as, say, Antimonium Tartaricum. However, knowing the cause, he may decide to begin therapy with the isopathic, and to prescribe cigarette smoke in potency, tacitly acknowledging the existence of a group disease.

The effect of the prescription will be to eliminate the essence of cigarette smoke from the body. Physical elimination may or may not follow, depending, in this example, on physical factors, though the essential healing will have already begun. That is the isopathic use of a potentialised medicine (the vector in potency), the use of which is reserved for a group disease. (Naturally, he could prescribe Antimonium Tartaricum, at the same time.)

Alternatively, to continue the example, the homoeopath might prescribe the potentised pathological product of smoker's bronchitis, i.e. the appropriate nosode. This type of remedy will be found useful not only to the patient but to all the members of the pathogenetic group.

In both cases—homoeotherapy and isotherapy—the practitioner must be able to source the remedy, and while this is a straightforward process in the case of the homoeopathic, the appropriate isopathic may prove to be more difficult to identify, and may have to be manufactured by the physician (though this would not be difficult to achieve, especially using radionics).

Autopathic solution

A third solution would be to potentise a sample of the patient himself, e.g. his sputum, and to create an autopathic (discussed in Chapter 4). This solution has the benefit that it assists the **entelechy** to allocate its own priorities.

HEALING PATTERNS

Primary detoxification

Detoxification should ideally be a first consideration, though there may be reason why this is postponed: usually because it is not urgently required, or because there is another, more urgent, matter to attend to. (See next chapter.)

Steady cure scenario

Usually, the homoeopath begins by prescribing for the individual homoeopathically, simply because palliation is required, then proceeds immediately to toxic elimination (of the group vector).

Alternatively, in the absence of apparent toxicity, the practitioner may decide to postpone detoxification. In any case, he will then move on to nosodal therapy in order to eliminate the influence of the pathogenetic group. As long as the pathogen has been identified that is a viable course.

The bond of the group disease will always be weakened at this stage. Supervening acute episodes may be dealt with homoeopathically.

Eventually, the patient will be free of the enrolling group, and will have been detoxified. He may then display for the first time the true symptoms of the disease state—typically, delusion will emerge—that caused him to attract the group vector in the first place. It is at this point that the possibility of relapse is defined. The patient will become a simple 'neurotic' case and may be treated as such homoeopathically.

Eventually, even that state will pass, and the patient may be treated as a relatively symptom-free constitution.

Underlying group disease scenario

The exception to steady cure is underlying group disease. In this scenario, the patient no sooner eliminates one group disease when another appears.

For example, a patient whose exposure to addictive substances began *in utero* may never become symptom-free, especially if there has been structural damage. If, for example, the patient's mother had been a substance addict during pregnancy, the case may prove to be unresolvable. In this case the correct approach would to address the *in utero* disturbance.

Given that the patient's susceptibility to certain types of group disease, for example, pulmonary diseases, will always be to some extent the result of the *in utero* disturbance, regardless of later aetiologies, e.g. smoking, it makes sense to prescribe to the primary group disease, in this case, the group disease of the mother. It is possible that the correct group disease prescription would remove the remaining symptomatology.

The general result

In general, what we observe in group disease prescribing is the elimination of group symptoms, including those associated with later secondary diseases, except where permanent physical damage prevents cure. That physical aftermath may or may not be reversible, or may cease to be a health issue.

Cases of dramatic and complete cure following the administration of a primary group disease isopathic may be observed in children who were healthy until they were vaccinated, when they permanently *ceased* to be healthy, a condition known as vaccinosis.

The standard homoeopathic approach to the primary group disease in these cases is to prescribe a single dose of the generic remedy Vaccininum, or a more specific aetiological nosode, e.g. DPT.

Residual group disease influence

Often, a remedy that is isopathic to an epidemic disease is prescribed in eliminating potencies after the bout of illness has subsided, especially if it is suspected that the disease has left an aftermath. Often this is done before or after the homoeopathic is prescribed, as a detoxification measure.

An isopathic nosode should be prescribed after an acute complaint has been treated homoeopathically and the acute symptoms have abated. (See Example Set 5.1).

If the disease is a form of environmental toxicity, and the toxin is no longer present in the patient's external environment, then the way is clear for isotherapy. If naturopathic detoxification has been completed, but residual toxicity is suspected, the correct step would be to prescribe isotherapeutically using the potentised group disease vector. (The procedures for this form of treatment are discussed in the next chapter.)

Even if there is no sign of physical toxicity, the group disease nosode may still be prescribed.

Example Set 5.1 Clearing of residual group disease influence

Ex.	*Indication*	*Prescription*
1	Aftermath of measles	Morbillinum 10M once
2	Aftermath of influenza	Influenzinum 1M once
3	Aftermath of rubella	Rubellinum 1M once

Homoeoprophylaxis

Homoeoprophylaxis may be more easily understood in the context of group disease theory, as most of the its applications are related to the anticipated presence of identified endemic and epidemic influences. Homoeoprophylaxis is the subject of Part 4.

CASE REVIEW

The review has five phases:

- ascertaining how the patient took the medicine
- ascertaining the results
- analysis
- fresh case taking, as required
- prescribing.

Broadly, the following results of prescribing can occur:

- amelioration
- aggravation followed by amelioration
- amelioration followed by relapse
- prolonged aggravation
- no change
- new symptoms

POSSIBLE PRESCRIBING OUTCOMES

Amelioration

If the potency was high enough to cause detoxification (but not high enough to cause toxic overload or proving), you should check for residual toxicity or a new symptom picture.

Aggravation followed by amelioration

Partial detoxification has occurred. Either the patient has adopted a lesser state of symptomatology or he has expelled the toxin completely, which is the less likely outcome.

Amelioration followed by relapse

The patient may need further exposures to the medicine at higher potencies.

If you prescribed an isopathic together with a homoeopathic, then the life force responded to a correctly selected remedy, and the patient then began to feel the beneficial effects of detoxification. Repeat the prescription with a higher potency of isopathic.

Isopathic aggravation

Isopathic aggravation is defined as an acute episode of toxicity following the administration of an isopathic, and is in fact an acute episode of the parent group disease. Palliation may be achieved with the similimum.

Whereas in homoeopathic prescribing, unexpected side effects of cure resulting from elimination of toxins may or may not occur, in isopathic prescribing side effects may be anticipated. Naturally, the more that is known about the original group disease the better.

Prolonged aggravation

This could mean that the patient is experiencing the side effects of detoxification, and may need palliation, or the prescription of supportive remedy, or both. Incidentally, elimination of vectors will be well under way.

No change
The potency was probably too low.

New symptoms
Assuming that the physician did not prescribe the similimum, the appearance of new symptoms usually results from using an isopathic that has never been subjected to a homoeopathic proving. Such symptoms may constitute new knowledge about the remedy, so a note should be made.

New symptoms could also appear when detoxification allows the symptom picture to clear, indicating an underlying condition.

ANTIDOTING

Note that the ill-effects of a remedy prescribed isopathically cannot be antidoted if they are due to the elimination of a toxic substance, as the remedy will need to run its course. As long as the toxin remains in the body, only palliation may be achieved with a homoeopathic. Moreover, curative prescribing will have to wait until a clear picture has emerged.

Note also that a homoeopathic cannot be used to antidote the harmful effects of a physical toxin—e.g. alcohol—that is causing illness, though it could be used to reduce the ill-effects themselves, e.g. hangover.

Example Set 5.2 illustrates how post-isopathic palliation—actually supportive prescribing—might be done. The first three examples assume that detoxification is required for a disease vectored by a microorganism, while the next three cases assume that toxicity is due to a non-biological influence.

Example Set 5.2 Post-isopathic palliation

Situation	*Isopathic*	*Homoeopathic palliative*
Shingles	Variolinum M	Rhus Toxicodendron 30C
Residual gonorrhoea symptoms	Medorrhinum 200C	Cubeba Officinalis 30X
Candida infection	Candida Albicans 12X	Lycopodium 30C
Nicotine toxicity	Nicotinum	Caladium Seguinum
Alcohol toxicity	Alcohol in potency	Nux Vomica
Cocaine toxicity	Cocainum	Avena Sativa

Whenever an isopathic has been administered, the assumption should be made that, provided the remedy was well selected, there will be a response. But because acute symptoms for the toxicity often have not been established, isopathic aggravation may be impossible to predict.

Note that any antidote which is given will not remove the essence of the isopathic, but might only palliate. That is because the elimination will have begun.

(These topics are the subject of Book 3 of the series.)

KEY DISTINCTIONS

Entelechy An organism's governing intelligence.

6 - ISOPATHIC DETOXIFICATION

INTRODUCTION
CLASSES OF TOXINS
Exotoxins
Endotoxins
BENEFITS OF DETOXIFICATION
DETOXIFICATION PROTOCOLS
THE ELIMINATION RESPONSE
DIRECT AND INDIRECT ELIMINATION
SUBSTANCE ABUSE
Effect on therapy
Management
DESIGNING A DETOXIFICATION STRATEGY
Contraindications for an elimination strategy
GEMMOTHERAPY

INTRODUCTION

Toxins are substances and influences within the diseased individual organism which indicate the presence of group disease. Within the morphogenetic disease group they act as disease vectors. Toxins are not limited to harmful environmental substances, but include any influences that can trigger an illness state or a spike in delusion, e.g. ideologies, beliefs, habits etc.

The organism is the vital force's organ of expression. Its natural tendency is to ingest and eliminate, rhythmically, and its systems of assimilation and elimination work together to that end. In illness that rhythm is always affected, causing the organism to compensate by, *inter alia*, absorbing and eliminating dysfunctionally. If necessary, it will generate its own disease products, e.g. pus, and eliminate *them*.

Toxins become obstacles to cure when the organism becomes overtaxed or damaged by them.

Homoeopathic detoxification (also referred to as drainage) is the elimination of toxins from the organism using potentialised medicines. Potentialised medicines will cause detoxification whether they are prescribed homoeopathically, as in routine homoeopathic prescribing, or isopathically, as in miasmatic prescribing. However, for strategic detoxification the prescription will be based on the remedy being prescribed isopathically.

CLASSES OF TOXINS

Toxins may be thought of as either **exotoxins** or **endotoxin**s. The distinction will have a bearing on treatment strategy.

Exotoxins

Exotoxins (or exogenous toxins) are substances and influences that are drawn into the organism in response to disturbance. They are commonly thought of as being only environmental toxic substances, allopathic drugs and recreational drugs, etc. However, they may also be thought of as including group disease vectors, e.g. toxins acquired during pregnancy, colonies of parasitic worms, internalised harmful ideologies, and so on.

The organism will unconsciously seek to draw in and retain exotoxins so that they may gravitate to their natural centre of disturbance. While the conscious decision to be healed will stop that tendency, the application of homoeopathic medicines will allow the flow to be reversed as cure occurs.

Note that isotherapy will result in detoxification without necessarily bringing about cure.

Endotoxins

Endotoxins (endogenous toxins) are substances or influences that are *generated by the organism* in response to disturbance. They include toxic pathological products, e.g. pus, fear and delusion, and inherited disease states.

The organism will unconsciously seek to release and eliminate endotoxins so that they may radiate to outer spheres. Like exotoxins, they may pool within the organism, especially if organs of elimination are weakened.

Toxic states may also be inherited, hence the hereditary group diseases, e.g. sickle-cell anaemia. Though inherited and self-generated toxins have been called autogenous toxins, the extra class is redundant, as all endogenous toxins may be thought of as being self-generated.

BENEFITS OF DETOXIFICATION

Detoxification:

- removes toxicosis that is obscuring the symptom picture and making it difficult to take a complete case

- removes substances and influences that are obstructing or retarding the work of homoeopathic medicines or of the natural tendency to self-heal
- removes substances and influences that tend to cause aggravations during homoeopathic treatment
- strengthens the immune system
- increases vital force
- increases the rate of repair of damaged tissues and organs
- assists metabolism.

DETOXIFICATION PROTOCOLS

The purpose of detoxification protocols is to assist the organism to eliminate toxins, including:

- allopathic drugs (see Chapter 7)
- industrial toxins
- recreational drugs
- toxic influences, e.g. iatrogenic psychiatry.

Detoxification will also be required to remove the by-products of:

- the metabolism of toxins
- tissue destruction caused by toxins.

THE ELIMINATION RESPONSE

All body systems are affected by detoxification, especially those which are actively involved in the elimination and storage of toxins, and those which may be passively affected, e.g. the nervous system. This is because the whole organism is involved in the initial disturbance, to which it responds in an attempt to minimise its discomfort by sacrificing its weakest tissues and organs. It will then re-experience some of this discomfort as it experiences healing. This effect is known as the ***elimination response***. This response may be anticipated, and treated homoeopathically (see *Designing a **detoxification strategy***, below).

Amplification of the vital force following the administration of an isopathic medicine often indicates the initiation of a slight eliminative proving, which may require a supportive homoeopathic. In fact, it would be unusual not to prescribe an isopathic without an adjunct homoeopathic, in anticipation of the side effects of elimination.

DIRECT AND INDIRECT ELIMINATION

Every remedy operates in the eliminative mode to some extent. However, this action is most pronounced when we prescribe the remedy for the primary purpose not of cure but of the elimination of toxicity, in other words, as part of an elimination strategy. In the eliminative mode physical elimination invariably occurs, and in the case of **indirect elimination** there may also be emotional discharge.

For the purpose of considering elimination strategies it is useful to distinguish between direct and indirect elimination:

- *Direct elimination*—achieved by the use of an isopathic and a homoeopathic together. The term *detoxification*, when used to refer to a prescribing strategy, usually refers to **direct elimination**.

- *Indirect elimination*—achieved by the use of a homoeopathic medicine alone, without targeting a particular toxin. Indirect elimination is the routinely observed by-product of homoeopathic cure.

SUBSTANCE ABUSE

Substance abuse is the excessive or addictive ingestion, inhalation, injection or absorption of any potentially toxic substance.

A small amount of any substance will act as a general stimulus to the organism, drawing increased expression from the life force. A small amount of a given toxin might have no influence on the curative process—it depends on the substance, the susceptibility of the patient and the remedy selected.

Depending on the substance, a slightly larger amount will cause general and particular dysfunction, and at a certain point of exposure saturation, chronicity will set in. Finally, massive ingestion will cause overwhelming structural damage to vital organs.

Addictive substances work rapidly on the nervous system to cause general primary symptoms and specific secondary symptoms. Each ingestion will result in a fresh bout of acute disease. As an addiction increases, so does related structural damage. In the end, whole body systems may become irreparably damaged.

The substance at the level of toxicity causes a sufficiently large disturbance of the organism to result in a distortion of the flow of the life force. That series of events is in itself a new disease—the group disease named after the specific substance being abused: cigarette abuse, carbohydrate abuse, and so on. The vector of the group disease is the substance itself, e.g. alcohol.

Effect on therapy

Substance abuse causes the total symptom picture to become clouded with the symptoms of the associated group disease. While that state is present, attempts to cure a chronic disease will fail.

Removal of the group disease will result in the second effect of substance abuse: immediate appearance of symptoms as the organism reacts to the withdrawal of the substance.

An addiction is a manifestation of a deep disturbance, so all of the spheres of human life become involved, beginning with general behaviour and the pains of cravings. If homoeopathic medicines have already been given in such a case, this stage may well prevent the medicines from working.

The third effect of substance abuse results from maintaining withdrawal of the addictive substance. The elimination process may cause a completely new symptom picture to emerge.

Management

Careful case taking will reveal any substance abuse that has occurred or that may be present. Often, there is a significant history of discontinued substance abuse, e.g. smoking. The patient may consider that there has been no aftermath, but there is always the possibility that the vital force has been permanently altered.

Current addictions need to be discontinued, if that is possible. Even before withdrawal, the very act of deciding to withdraw will cause symptoms of apprehensiveness, craving, etc. If so, then you should prescribe homoeopathically for the acute state. Isopathic detoxification may then proceed.

DESIGNING A DETOXIFICATION STRATEGY

The use of a detoxification strategy is a way of relieving the ill-effects of having ingested a harmful substance, while preparing the patient for curative homoeopathic treatment, all the while protecting him from iatrogenic side effects.

Table 6.1 Suggested detoxification combinations

Case	*Purpose*	*Formula*
1	Indirect elimination	The appropriate homoeopathic followed by the appropriate homoeopathic in the event of an elimination response
2	Direct elimination of a specific toxin	A higher potency isopathic (vital force permitting) together with a lower potency homoeopathic, e.g. Berberis, in low potency, e.g. 6X
3	Direct elimination of a specific allergen	A lower potency isopathic together with a lower potency homoeopathic, eg Arsenicum Album 6C, or both
4	Direct elimination of a specific systemic toxin in the complete absence of acute symptoms and following homoeopathic treatment	The constitutional (if known) in a higher potency (vital force permitting) followed by the appropriate homoeopathic, should there be an elimination response
5	Indirect elimination and anticipation of specific organ stress	The constitutional (if known) in a higher potency (vital force permitting) together with a lower potency supportive remedy

Most detoxification strategies rely on a combinatorial approach, i.e. two medicines being prescribed simultaneously:

- an ***initiator*** *(or elimination) remedy* (the remedy of higher potency)
- a ***support*** *(or protective) remedy* (the remedy of lower potency).

Together, they form a ***detoxification combination***. The remedies are usually prescribed as simplexes, which gives maximum control over the adjustment of dosage.

Typically, the patient in need of detoxification requires first, isotherapy and, if that is successful, the constitutional. However, this is entirely in the hands of the practitioner, who may simply decide to make the similimum do all the work (and good luck to him on that score).

Your preference for a support remedy should be based on your perception of the weakest area of the organism, i.e. the organ or system most likely to require support when elimination increases. You may also decide to prescribe a complex of support medicines.

Regardless of the protocol adopted, you can expect the patient to get sick, and that is when the similimum will come into its own.

Table 6.1 contains some suggested formulae for detoxification combinations.

Contraindications for an elimination strategy

Caution is advised when the possible effect of an elimination strategy might be to induce elimination into the bloodstream of a dangerous or undesired substance, resulting in an unwanted *non-curative* aggravation, or proving (see Example Set 6.1).

Example Set 6.1 Contraindications for isopathics

Ex.	*Scenario*	*Contraindicated remedy*
1	History of cannabis addiction	Cannabis indica
2	History of lead poisoning	Plumbum metallicum
3	Side effects of methylphenidate used to control ADHD	Methylphenidate in potency

GEMMOTHERAPY

Gemmotherapy is the prescription of very low potency (Ø & 1D) phytotherapeutics manufactured from buds as glycerin macerates. Qua gemmotherapeutics they are prescribed on clinical indications alone, and are designed to act as detoxification agents, either alone or with other homoeopathics (see Example Set 6.2). Many of the series—there are 38 in all—are established homoeopathics.

Example Set 6.2 Gemmotherapeutics

Ex.	*Gemmotherapeutic*	*Deconcentration*	*Indication*
1	Abies Pectinata (Fir buds)	1D	Decalcification Rickets Dental caries
2	Taraxacum Officinale (Dandelion buds)	Ø	Constipation
3	Viscum Album (Mistletoe young shoots)	1D	Epilepsy Low blood pressure Metrorrhagia Retained placenta Ovaralgia Sciatica Muscular fibrillation

KEY DISTINCTIONS

Detoxification combination A combination of (usually two) medicines used in a detoxification strategy, consisting of: an *initiator (or elimination) remedy* (the remedy prescribed in the higher potency) and a *support (or protective) remedy* (the remedy prescribed in the lower potency). These *concurrent remedies* are prescribed as two separate simplexes, giving control over the adjustment of dosage.

Detoxification strategy A plan for detoxifying a patient, typically involving the prescription of a *detoxification combination* together with appropriate supporting measures, e.g. lifestyle adjustment.

Direct elimination **1.** Elimination that is achieved by the use of isotherapy and homoeotherapy together **2.** Detoxification, when used as a deliberate strategy.

Elimination response An increase in the elimination of toxins, often accompanied by symptoms.

Endotoxin Endogenous toxin. Substance or influence that is generated by the organism in response to disturbance. Endotoxins include mental and physical pathological products.

Exotoxin Exogenous toxin. A substance or influence that has been drawn into the organism in response to disturbance.

Gemmotherapy The use of low potency (Ø & 1D) phytotherapeutics manufactured from buds and prescribed on clinical indications alone, as agents of detoxification.

Indirect elimination The elimination of toxins which is routinely achieved as a by-product of homoeotherapy.

Initiator remedy In a detoxification combination, the remedy prescribed in the higher potency, usually an isopathic designed to initiate and maintain elimination of a group disease vector.

Support remedy In a detoxification combination, the remedy prescribed in the lower potency, usually for the support and protection of organs of elimination.

7 - IATROGENIC DISORDERS

INTRODUCTION
Categories
Chronic presentation
Acute presentation
Political abuse of medicine
EFFECTS ON THE VITAL FORCE
Pseudo-constitution
CASE TAKING
Medication history
Surgical procedures
Additional history
TREATMENT STRATEGY
Detoxification
Vaccinosis
When to use a homoeopathic
How to use an isopathic
DISCONTINUING PRESCRIBED MEDICATION
Necessary medication
Unnecessary medication

INTRODUCTION

Iatrogenic disorders are encountered routinely in homoeopathic medicine. Most, if not all, allopathic medical procedures either cause harmful side effects or suppress symptoms. Some of these effects may not be completely reversed, but most of them will be amenable to amelioration.

(It should go without saying that the necessary prescription of anaesthetics, analgesics, antibiotics, medication designed to preserve life, and so on, is *not* what this chapter is about, though common presentations sometimes include their residual or side effects, which are often unavoidable, and often can be addressed.)

Categories

In most, if not all such cases, allopathic physicians will be careful to minimise suffering, and will explain to the patient any difficulties to be expected.

The justification given by the prescribers of suppressive medication is that their chronic side effects (which may include a hastening of death) are generally outweighed by the mitigation of acute symptoms, which may not in themselves be as serious.

Where physicians do not explain the exact nature of the risk, or wrongly minimise or discount the risk of iatrogenic disorder, an additional class of disease may result. The iatrogenic disorders most commonly encountered by the homoeopathic physician may be classified by cause as follows:

- medical procedures designed to prevent the contraction or expression of a disease
- medical or surgical treatment designed to 'normalise' or 'standardise' a patient who is not ill, e.g. an autistic
- pharmacological, e.g. suppressive medication
- radiational
- institutional care
- wrong wellbeing management advice

- surgical, especially when unnecessary, or when designed to prevent the expression of disease
- political programmes designed to degrade the health status of subjects—fluoridation, vaccination, etc.
- political and state-approved (and parental-approved) forms of physical or mental force or restraint, including being irradiated, electrified, cut, burnt, poisoned, tortured or incarcerated, by or with the complicity of a physician.

Chronic presentation

Medication is suppressive when it is prescribed antipathically, i.e. to prevent symptoms. It will be apparent that all of the beneficial effects of allopathic medicine are included in that definition. That is because at best allopathic medicine is still a compromise, even though it is a compromise that we would all gladly make in the appropriate circumstances. Where the problem usually occurs is when the patient's experience of allopathic medicine is distressing. In those circumstances, he will benefit from esoteric medicine, which has as its principal aim the safe conduction of harmful or suppressed energy.

Acute presentation

To a lesser extent, the patient who has benefited greatly from allopathic medicine, but has been left with a slight or temporary aftermath—illness after anaesthetic, pain after surgery, nausea after radiotherapy, etc—will often be seen. Many of these cases are easy to prescribe to, and may even be anticipated (see Example Set 7.1).

Example Set 7.1 Solutions to acute iatrogenic disorders

Ex.	*Disorder*	*Prescription*	*Use of potency*
1	Ill-effects of radiotherapy	Cadmium Sulphuratum 30C	Homoeopathic
		Ipecacuanha 6C	Homoeopathic
2	Ill-effects of EEG using stroboscope	Cicuta Virosa 30C	Homoeopathic
		Rescue Remedy (Bach)	Homoeopathic
		Lux Stroboscopus 1M	Isopathic
3	Ill-effects of antibiotics	Penicillinum IM	Isopathic
4	Ill-effects of cancer diagnosis	Mimulus (Bach)	Homoeopathic
		Rescue Remedy (Bach)	Homoeopathic
		Mezereum	Homoeopathic

Political abuse of medicine

Any medical procedure that is ordered by the state (often with the complicity of parents) is iatrogenic, regardless of the reason, for the simple reason that the state cannot practise loving medicine. I say nothing about its necessary foundation in and maintenance by agents of inhumanity.

EFFECTS ON THE VITAL FORCE

Suppressive medication causes the flow of the vital force to change, with the result that the target symptoms may be mitigated, but only at the expense of the function of one of the vital organs, invariably the one most susceptible to destabilising in that individual. The result will be a diminution of the life force the organism needs for it to thrive.

However, suppressive medication often enables patients to make life choices they could not otherwise make (see Example

Set 7.2). Therefore, your task as a vitalistic physician is simply to indicate the possibilities, both for cure and for palliation.

Example Set 7.2 Suppressive medication

Ex.	*Drug*	*Medical Application*
1	Paracetamol	Pain control
2	Sodium valproate	Petit mal epilepsy
3	Insulin	Diabetes mellitus
4	BCG vaccination	None

Pseudo-constitution

Eventually, the suppressive medication will cause a distortion of the constitution itself. The problem is that, in some way the constitution lends itself to every symptom, so iatrogenic distortion should never be assumed to be superficial. Thus, if suppressive medication is reduced, any pseudo-constitution that has been created will tend to evaporate, revealing the true constitution.

CASE TAKING

Medication history

A complete medication history should be taken, including:

- over-the-counter medication
- antibiotics
- anaesthetics
- vaccination
- hormone therapy
- emergency medication, e.g. antivenin
- permanent medication, e.g. anticonvulsants

- emergency medication, e.g. puffers
- psychotropic medication
- oral contraceptives.

You will need to ascertain:

- what medication the patient is currently taking and whether he needs it
- whether he has ever stopped taking it and what happened
- what side effects, if any, he has experienced
- modalities for the side effects, e.g. > lying down
- whether the patient drinks alcohol, smokes cannabis, etc.
- whether the patient has ever had an adverse reaction to any medication
- whether the patient has any allergies or sensitivities.

Surgical procedures

All surgical and invasive examination procedures result in iatrogenic disorder, either directly, e.g. because they are distressing or cause an inflammatory response, or because they involve premedication or medication, e.g. general anaesthetic, or both, e.g. epidural block. Many of these procedures have traditionally attracted classic remedy responses, some of which appear in Example Set 7.3.

Additional history

Patients who complain of the aftermath of medical procedures should be asked to describe their experience and understanding of the procedures experienced by them, and their current physical or emotional experience. Occasionally, a patient will have had a long series of related or similar experiences, especially if he has a long history of serious illness.

Example Set 7.3 Surgical & invasive examination procedures

Ex.	*Procedure*	*Prescription*
1	Inguinal hernia repair	Strontium Carbonicum 30C four times a day
2	Radiotherapy	Nux Vomica 30C hourly, if necessary
3	Endoscopy	Silica 30X four times a day
4	Dental filling (and its anticipation)	Hypericum 10M four times a day
5	Eye surgery	Ruta Graviolens 10X hourly

TREATMENT STRATEGY

The following might be discussed with the patient:

- side effects and dangers of over-the-counter medication, prescribed medication and recreational drugs
- any side effects that you or the patient may have observed
- the possibilities of homoeopathic prescribing
- the options for support you can offer, including communication with the patient's doctor
- how you propose to manage the patient's shift to homoeopathic medicines
- the need to maintain necessary prescribed medication for the time being
- drug manufacturers' recommendations, especially regarding discontinuing prescribed medication.

Detoxification

In the long term, homoeopathic detoxification will be required if the patient has symptoms that are suspected of having arisen out of any of the following:

- vaccination
- general anaesthetics
- antibiotic therapy
- hormone therapy
- cancer chemotherapy
- other chemotherapy
- psychotropic drugs
- non-steroidal anti-inflammatory drugs (NSAIDS) and opioids.

On the other hand, an allopathic drug may do its work so well that the patient is prevented from displaying the symptoms it prevents. The symptom picture will become clearer—and less confused—as the patient:

- takes supportive measures, e.g. corrects his diet
- discontinues over-the-counter orthodox medication
- discontinues self-prescribed alternative medicines
- discontinues optional prescribed medication
- discontinues recreational drugs
- adjusts his lifestyle: sleeps more, exercises correctly, avoids stressful situations, etc.

Table 7.4 illustrates how the problem may be approached, though the possible presentations are endless, and the examples are not definitive. For contrast, I have included several solutions that are purely homoeopathic (marked with an asterisk).

Vaccinosis

The removal of the ill-effects of vaccination and vaccine toxins—formaldehyde, mercury, aluminium phosphate, detergent, paraffin oil, bacteria etc—have been mentioned. Example Set 7.5 shows the various classes of vaccinosis remedies. The standard approach, as always, is to lead with a homoeopathic whenever the patient is sick.

Example Set 7.4 Detoxification solutions

Ex.	*Scenario*	*Possible solution*
1	Generalised hypersensitivity	Sepia 1M*
2	Mercury ingestion following amalgam replacement	Mercurius 30C + Berberis 30C
3	House dust allergy	House dust 3C + Adrenalinum 3C
4	Long history of cannabis smoking	Cannabis Indica 6C + Chamomilla 30C
5	Cigarette withdrawal is accompanied by gastrointestinal symptoms	Cigarette 3C + Caladium Seguinum 30C
6	All attempts at detoxification cause pungent smelling sweat	Mercurius Solubilis 1M+ Pyrogenium 12C*
7	Highly robust male with long history of ingestion of Ritalin	Ritalin 6C + Belladonna 200C
8	Child never well since ingestion of prescribed methylphenidate	Concerta 6LM + Calcarea Carbonica 1M
9	Autism < following vaccination	Pertussinum + Silicea
10	Alcoholism	Quercus Pedunculata (Gemmotherapeutic) 1DH*

*These are purely homoeopathic solutions.

When to use a homoeopathic

The similimum should be used in the presence of frank symptoms that indicate it. A number of these have been found to be particularly effective for this use. In general, the more specific symptoms are, the more likely a homoeopathic will appear. And, as always, the constitutional will tend to bring out symptoms that are indefinite, but noticed—usually by the mother.

Example Set 7.5 Classes of vaccinosis remedies

Ex.	*Remedy*	*Class*	*Remedy action*	*Application*
1	Mezereum	Similar	Homoeopathic	General
2	Silicea	Similar	Homoeopathic	General
3	Thuja Occidentalis	Similar	Homoeopathic	General
4	Vaccininum	Generic	Isopathic	General
5	Diphtherinum	Specific	Isopathic	Diphtheria
6	Pertussinum	Specific	Isopathic	Whooping cough
7	Tetaninum	Specific	Isopathic	Tetanus

How to use an isopathic

Naturally, when prescribing isopathically the best results will be obtained by administering the actual vaccine used in potency, instead of the generic. There are two reasons for this: first, the vaccine will contain other toxins in addition to the vaccine product, e.g. adjuvants and preservatives, and second, the vaccine may contain a combination of pathogenic products and toxoids, e.g. several different influenza viruses.

One solution is to potentise the actual product, which may be obtained by the patient with an allopathic prescription, and will ensure a closer isopathic match. This is easily done with a potency simulator, or using the Korsakovian method.

Potencies used to deal with the ill-effects of vaccination should be commensurate with the vital force, which will usually be low and, in the case of children, may benefit from being high-phase, indicating the 50-millesimal potency (see Chapter 11 of Book 1).

The generic group disease isopathic, Vaccininum, has also been found by the author to be particularly effective, as have the various vaccines in potency.

(See also Example Set 7.6.)

Example Set 7.6 Typical vaccinosis solutions

Ex.	*Situation*	*Prescription*	*Frequency of repetition*
1	Side effects of recent DPT vaccination	A complex: Diphtherinum 1LM, Pertussinum 1LM and Tetaninum 1LM	Once a day for a week
2	Side effects of recent DPT vaccination	Vaccininum 1LM	Once a day for a week
3	Side effects of recent DPT vaccination	Silicea 4LM	3 times a day for a week
4	Autism following vaccination	Thuja Occidentalis 4LM	Once a day for 2 weeks
5[1]	Anticipated unspecified side effects of Rubella vaccination	Rubellinum 1LM	Once a day for a week
6[1]	Anticipated specific side effects of vaccination	Calcarea Carbonica 6C	Once a day for a week

1. As usual, potencies prescribed in anticipation of ill-effects of vaccination should be kept low. Apart from the fact that the low potency will be a precaution against a proving, it is in keeping with the general rule that an uncertain symptomatology will not merit a confident potency level.

DISCONTINUING PRESCRIBED MEDICATION

A patient may have issues surrounding the proposed withdrawal of allopathically prescribed medication, even completely unnecessary medication, and the subject may need to be addressed with sensitivity. Also, any concerns the patient may have about homoeopathic medication will also need to be addressed. This will especially be the case when the prospect of withdrawal causes anxiety and actual withdrawal causes severe symptoms—even if they are not life-threatening—as in many psychiatric disorders.

Necessary medication

A patient should not discontinue necessary prescribed medication, e.g. life supporting medication or medication that suppresses severe manifestations—psychosis, epilepsy, and so on. However, you may prescribe a homoeopathic simultaneously; normally this would present no problem. The following steps would then be taken:

1. Discuss your strategy with the patient.
2. Prescribe homoeopathically to the presenting picture, beginning with low potencies. (Do not begin isopathic detoxification while the patient continues to eliminate the toxin spontaneously.)
3. Explain to the patient that he could experience the symptoms of an overdose of his prescribed *allopathic* medication if as healing occurs and that he must discuss

this possibility with the prescriber. It might be necessary to write a note to this effect for the other physician.

4. Do not ask the patient to discontinue his medication without seeking advice from the prescriber.
5. Review often, by telephone if necessary.

Unnecessary medication

Should the patient decide to discontinue non-essential prescribed medication or medication that is not designed to support the life force, you should:

- advise the patient about the effects of the medication and of its withdrawal
- treat the patient homoeopathically
- if the allopathic medication has had the effect of preventing a symptom picture from emerging, consider homoeopathic detoxification
- ask the patient not to discontinue his medication without seeking advice from the prescriber.

8 - ISOPATHIC POTENCY SELECTION

PRESCRIBING SCENARIOS
Aetiology
Allergic and hypersensitivity reactions
Autopathy
Concurrent medication
Constitutional
The potency of the constitutional
Detoxification
Homoeopathic detoxification
Isopathic detoxification
Autopathic detoxification
Elimination
Epidemic prescribing
Euthenic prescribing
Group disease and miasmatic prescribing
Iatrogenic disorders
Prophylaxis
Vaccinosis
CHAPTER SUMMARY

PRESCRIBING SCENARIOS

This chapter suggests practical **potency selection** solutions in specific areas of prescribing. (Readers might consider reviewing Book 1, Chapter 10, if they have not already done so.)

This is a synoptic chapter, not a chapter on therapeutics, so it is not meant to be definitive. Also, the list of possible scenarios is not meant to be exhaustive.

Several of these scenarios also suggest homoeopathic options (briefly discussed in Book 1, Chapter 8).

Aetiology

A known aetiology that is not identifiable with an event (or series of events), e.g. a motor vehicle accident, but is the result of some form of exposure or contagion, is a case for isopathic treatment, e.g. an elimination strategy (whether by itself or with a homoeopathic), as there will always be a definite vector (see Example Set 8.1).
(See also *Group disease and miasmatic prescribing*, below.)

Example Set 8.1 Aetiological prescribing (isopathic)

Ex.	*Presentation*	*Aetiology*	*Prescription*
1	Chronic fatigue syndrome	Infectious mononucleosis	Epstein-Barr virus in potency + Phosphoricum Acidum 30C
2	Hepatitis C	Needle sharing	Hepatitis C nosode in potency + Pyrogenium 30C
3	Oophoritis	Suppression of gonorrhoea	Medorrhinum 200C + Colocynthis 30C

Allergic and hypersensitivity reactions

Generally, if a patient requests treatment for allergy, is able to identify the allergen, *and is asymptomatic*, treatment may be carried out isopathically. The treatment for a *specific* allergy is actually a form of hyposensitisation. In hyposensitisation an isopathic is usually prescribed at a low numerical potency on a small scale, sometimes with a supporting remedy. (See Example Set 8.2.)

Example Set 8.2 Allergic and hypersensitivity reactions

Ex.	*Scenario*	*Prescription*
1	Pollen hyposensitisation programme	1st month: Pollen 6X + Adrenalinum 3X 2nd month: Pollen 9X + Adrenalinum 3X 3rd month: Pollen 12X + Adrenalinum 3X
2	House dust hyposensitisation programme	1st month: House Dust 3X + Histaminum 3X 2nd month: House Dust 6X + Histaminum 3X 3rd month: House Dust 9X + Histaminum 3X
3	Allergic rhinitis (due to coffee) with intervening (unrelated) allergic reaction	1st Month: Coffea 3X + Euphrasia 6X On development of urticaria after eating strawberries: Oxalicum Acidum 6C until resolved Resume coffee hyposensitisation

If the patient has a history of asthma or anaphylactic shock, treatment should only be performed homoeopathically, and at a higher potency, e.g. 24X. Also, should a patient present with allergic symptoms or become symptomatic during hyposensitisation, any treatment given from that point until the subsidence of symptoms should be homoeopathic (i.e. not isopathic). Note that in Example 3 the intervening reaction is due to an unrelated event.

Autopathy

As discussed in Chapter 4, prescribing a potentialised medicine made from the patient's own body (sometimes from an effected part) has a long history, both in detoxification (see below) and therapy generally, though the results are unpredictable.

It is considered that a higher potency concurrent homoeopathic, possibly the constitutional, might also be appropriate, depending on the circumstances.

See Example Set 8.3.

Example Set 8.3 Autopathic prescribing

Ex.	*Complaint*	*Prescription*	*Frequency*
1	Alopecia	Patient's head hair 3C	q.i.d until >
2	Effects of grief	Lacriminum (Patient's tears) 3C	q.i.d. until >
3	Herpes zoster	Salivinum (Patient's saliva 3C)	q.i.d. until >

Concurrent medication

When prescribing two remedies concurrently it is recommended that the numerical potencies be widely different, thereby separating the energy levels being addressed. The remedies will then have separate spheres of action. Medicines that are based on edible plants, e.g. Calendula, often will be found to be quite gentle in low potencies. (See Example Set 8.4.)

Occasionally, the lower of two concurrent potencies will be homoeopathic when the other is an isopathic. In that case, the prescriber should ensure that the homoeopathic will exert a suitably *protective* effect, in anticipation of detoxification. This may be achieved by selecting homoeopathics that are associated with disorders of the eliminative organs.

Experience and a knowledge of toxicology and symptomatology will assist in the choice of a remedy.

(See also *Remedy Multiplicity* in Book 2, Chapter 9.)

Example Set 8.4 Concurrent medication

Ex.	*Situation*	*Prescription*
1	Detoxification before and after dental amalgam replacement	Mercurius Solubilis 1M + Phytolacca 30C
2	Gonorrhoea	Sulphur 200C + Cubeba Officinalis 12X
3	Candidiasis	Candida Albicans 200X + Lycopodium 30C
4	Facial impetigo	Antimonium Tartaricum + Viola Tricolor

Constitutional

There are four circumstances in which one might consider prescribing the known or apparent constitutional:

- to encourage symptoms when the vital force has settled at a low point
- to encourage symptoms when the vital force has been suppressed
- to encourage vitality when symptoms have been dispelled, but the patient is still not well
- to maintain health post-therapeutically.

The following are some typical prescribing scenarios. Examples of possible prescriptions for the following scenarios are shown in Example Set 8.5: Constitutional prescribing.

Scenario 1

The patient is ill but not showing clear symptoms beyond general symptoms that are too vague to prescribe on, e.g. irritableness, lethargy, etc. The practitioner wishes to cause the vital force to expand, causing it to express the latent symptoms, so that he may discover the similimum. It will not be necessary to later antidote the effects of the constitutional. The potency level should be higher than the vital force would seem to require. Dosage should be frequent until symptoms are manifested.

Scenario 2

The patient's life force has been suppressed *generally*, and there are no specific new or recent symptoms. This is the usual situation at the end of a long period of illness, especially one in which there may have been a high degree of artificial suppression, e.g. cancer. The potency level should be higher than the vital force would seem to require. Dosage should be frequent. Note that if you suspect that iatrogenic suppression has occurred, you should anticipate the spontaneous release of symptomatogenic essences and, perhaps, substances.

Scenario 3

The patient has successfully completed a course of homoeotherapy and is free of symptoms. The constitutional will increase the radiant inclination of expression, causing amplification of the individual's characteristic life force and general amelioration. As long as the patient remains well, he may continue to take the remedy occasionally.

The potency of the constitutional

Note that constitutionals are polychrests, those being the only remedies that have the breadth of action to match the classically recognised constitutional diatheses. Even so, each possesses its own unique intrinsic vital force, which may be activated by the appropriate level of potentisation. Some, e.g. Phosphorus, may require only a low potency to bring out their best, while others, e.g. Ignatia, may require a higher potency.

Example Set 8.5 Constitutional prescribing

Scenario	*Situation*	*Prescription*
1	Vital force has settled at a low point	Sepia 30C
2	Vital force has been artificially suppressed	Natrum Muriaticum 1M
3	Symptoms have *apparently* been dispelled	Phosphorus 10C

(See also Book 1, Chapter 7: *Constitution and diathesis*, and Chapter 15: *Constitutional prescribing*, and Book 2, *passim*.)

Detoxification

Isopathic detoxification

It should be noted that the healing gradient should be designed to facilitate only the degree of response required to conduct the group disease vectors and influences away from the patient, harmlessly. A greater gradient than is required may result in a sudden increase in toxicity owing to the body's inability to be rid of it, causing an aggravation.

On the other hand, a healing gradient that is insufficient will result in a failure to eradicate the symptomatology.

The remedy selected unwisely will, of course, cause the organism to conduct the isopathic essence and substance, and may also result in the patient displaying the symptoms of a proving, i.e. new and additional symptoms.

Most detoxification techniques involve giving the patient an isopathic together with a homoeopathic, in widely differing potencies.

In isopathy, we are dealing with group disease, and the organism is treated as the representative of the group, i.e. the individual's host social group, race or species. For that reason, the higher attenuations have been found to be efficacious, not because of any scalar advantage—potency packaging offers none—but due to the high number of succussions used to produce a high potency.

Example Set 8.6 Detoxification

Ex.	*Situation*	*Prescription*	*Frequency of Repetition*
1	Candidiasis	Candida Albicans 1M (Isopathic) + Taraxacum 30C (hepatoprotective)	Both medicines three times a day for one month
2	Cigarette withdrawal	Caladium 30C (homoeopathic) + Chelidonium 6X (hepatoprotective)	Both medicines three times a day for two weeks
3	Heroin addiction	Opium 1M (homoeopathic) + Avena Sativa 30C (hepatoprotective)	Both medicines three times a day for two weeks
4	Urinary tract infection	Cannabis Sativa M + Auto-urine 6LM (Korsakovian)	Both medicines once a day for a week

The higher potency will create a steep elimination gradient in a more central sphere for the vital force and cause symptoms to be expressed. The lower potency, which may be prescribed prophylactically, will provide a more gentle healing gradient to allow the vital force to express any disturbance that, as the result of the higher potency, it might experience in a more external, e.g. organic, sphere. Examples of prescriptions are shown in Example Set 8.6.

Homoeopathic detoxification

All homoeotherapy results in elimination of some kind, which might be more or less significant, depending on the aetiology. Thus, the similimum should not be thought of as having the primary function of an eliminator.

In this book special detoxification using potentised remedies should be taken to mean isopathy.

Autopathic detoxification

Potencies should be started low, regardless of the vital force, as autopathics often have a dramatic effect. (See also Book 2, Chapter 8.)

Elimination

Elimination is discussed elsewhere (see Chapter 6) in relation to allergy, hyposensitisation, detoxification, euthenic therapy, and miasm. Of course, in most cases, what is meant by elimination is elimination of toxins. The most important fact to bear in mind is that cure is accompanied by elimination. Indeed, one could say that elimination is the measure of cure. Elimination will therefore be at its most complex and interesting during homoeotherapy. And given that the patient's level of vitality is bound to increase as cure proceeds, one can expect to finish therapy with a high potency.

Epidemic prescribing

During an epidemic it is permissible to prescribe isopathically for the elimination of the group disease vector, and his may be done in conjunction with homoeotherapy. Homoeopathic potencies are usually selected to match the patient's vitality, except when prescribing prophylactically, when it is permissible to prescribe *in anticipation* of the patient's level of vitality. (See Example Set 8.7.)

Example Set 8.7 Epidemic prescribing

Ex.	*Situation*	*Prescription*	*Frequency of repetition*
1	Mumps recurrence	Parotidinum IM + Baryta Carbonica 3LM	Hourly until improved
2	Anticipation of measles	Morbillinum 1M + Pulsatilla 1LM	Once a day for one week
3	Influenza	Influenzinum 1M + Eupatorium Perfoliatum 12C	Twice a day until improved

(See also *Prophylaxis,* below).

Euthenic prescribing

In euthenic therapy, the aim is to detoxify the patient or remove noxious influences (classical: miasms) — sometimes both.

Example Set 8.8 Euthenic prescribing

Ex.	*Situation*	*Prescription*	*Roles of medicines*
1	Previous addiction	Cigarette 1M + Caladium 30C[1]	Isopathic + homoeopathic
2	Cause of mother's death	Tuberculinum 30C	Isopathic
3	Previous group disease	Rubellinum 30C	Isopathic

1. Homoeopathic supportive

As discussed in Chapter 4, potencies can be used to detoxify the pregnant patient who has had or currently has a group disease, e.g. cigarette addiction, or even if there are grounds for suspecting the presence of a group disease, e.g. where there is a family history of a disease. The disease might take the form of a hereditary disease or disease diathesis, e.g. pulmonary weakness.

The mother to be can be medicated serially with the group disease in potency during the first trimester, once a week for each isopathic. Several examples are shown in Example Set 8.8. Of course, it would be preferable if this preparation could be undertaken *before* pregnancy began.

Group disease and miasmatic prescribing

Where there is evidence that the symptomatology has been dominated by an old group toxicity, e.g. malaria, the correct purification procedure is to give the appropriate elimination remedy in a potency calculated to facilitate the unimpeded flow of vital force. (See Example Set 8.9.)

Example Set 8.9 Group disease and miasmatic prescribing

Ex.	*Situation*	*Prescription*	*Frequency*
1	History of chicken pox	Variolinum 30C	Daily until >
2	History of cancer	Carcinosinum 10M	Weekly until >
3	Persistent symptoms following scarlet fever	Scarlatininum 1M + Ammonium Carbonicum 1LM	Daily until >

The seriousness of the consequences of the particular group illness will give an indication of the depth of the disturbance. Thus, we would regard the childhood illnesses as a family as being less deep than the malignancies. (See also *Epidemic prescribing* and *Vaccinosis*.)

Iatrogenic disorders

See Chapter 7.

Prophylaxis

For general guidelines relating to the selection of potency for homoeoprophylaxis for medical procedures, epidemic prescribing, group disease (and miasmatic prescribing), obstetrics, ordeal, travelling and vaccination, see Chapter 10.

Vaccinosis

See *Treatment Strategy: Vaccinosis* in Chapter 7.

CHAPTER SUMMARY

Generally, homoeopathic solutions are a much simpler business than isopathics, where there will be certain elimination, usually requiring a concurrent homoeopathic. In those cases it will be necessary to calibrate two potencies at once, usually a high (leading) potency, and the other a lower (protective or supportive) potency.

When the patient has a disease requiring some form of physical detoxification, the homoeopathic element—the protective—is far more likely to produce a recognisable proving in a high enough potency, and may be controlled more easily.

When the patient has a group disease in the classical miasmic sense, i.e. one that is generally regarded as contagious, the patient may usually be given high potencies, simply because they already have a proving in progress.

In both cases, the second remedy—assuming an iso-homoeopathic strategy—will be prescribed in a widely separate potency.

KEY CONCEPTS

Posology The study of dosage. In homoeopathy it is concerned solely with the measure of the patient's exposure to the remedy.

Potency selection The creation of a potency that will match the patient's resistance to the flow of the vital force, thereby annihilating it.

PART 4
HOMOEOPATHIC PROPHYLAXIS

9 Approach to homoeopathic prophylaxis
10 Homoeopathic prophylaxis in practice

9 - APPROACH TO HOMOEOPATHIC PROPHYLAXIS

INTRODUCTION
PRINCIPLE MODES OF APPLICATION
Prophylaxis not preventive
Key symptom anticipation
Possible curative effect
Action
THE HOMOEOPROPHYLAXIS MYTHOS
Immunity
Advance cure
PRESCRIBING PROTOCOLS
The isopathic protocol (isoprophylaxis)
Epidemic prophylaxis
Group disease
Travelling
The homoeopathic protocol (homoeoprophylaxis)
Generic illness
Medical procedure
Ordeal
The iso-homoeopathic protocol (iso-homoeoprophylaxis)
VACCINATION

INTRODUCTION

Homoeopathic prophylaxis, or homoeoprophylaxis, may be more easily understood in the context of group disease theory, as most of its applications are related to the intuited or anticipated presence of identified endemic and epidemic influences. In that sense, therefore, it is a branch of isopathy.

Note, however, that, though there are in reality two common prophylactic protocols (isopathic and homoeopathic), they are usually used together.

PRINCIPLE MODES OF APPLICATION

Prophylaxis not preventive

The aim of prophylaxis is to install persistent susceptibility in anticipation of a disturbance of the vital force, thereby facilitating the eventual harmless conduction of the anticipated group disease influence (*not* to prevent disease).

Thus, the prophylactic application exploits the *susceptive* mode of medicinal response in order to achieve its apparent delayed protective effect. (See Chapters 9-10 of Book 1.)

Key symptom anticipation

While potentialised medicines are usually used to reduce *existing* illness, prophylactic prescribing is used when the key indicator, or 'symptom', is *anticipation of illness (*either generic or specific), which is a clear indication that the presence of a group disease influence has been intuited by the patient.

Possible curative effect

The minimising effect of the prophylactic is indicated by the *familiar* anticipated threat to the individual, and not to any extant pathology of the individual (though, like the homoeopathic, isopathic, and constitutional, the prophylactic may have a curative effect in the event of it turning out to be the actual similimum to a latent, or perhaps historical, morphogenetic field influence, which would be a bonus).

Its actual curative effect is on the level of the related familiar morphogenetic field, whose influence it will weaken. Any transient apparent proving which may occur in the patient will be due to the installation and maintenance (by serial medications) of the prophylactic's healing gradient, and may be regarded as analogous to the homoeopathic aggravation.

Action

The idea behind giving a prophylactic is to install a healing gradient in anticipation of the patient's vital force subscribing to a particular group disease, e.g. influenza. The net result of the interaction of the prophylactic and the disease will be, at least, a lessening of the severity of the disease, and at best, a complete neutralisation of the disease state before it becomes frankly symptomatic.

THE HOMOEOPROPHYLAXIS MYTHOS

It follows from the foregoing that homoeoprophylaxis is not an attempt or programme to prevent disease. Disease cannot be completely prevented—the causative factors are far too mysterious. Attempts to bring about wellbeing will minimise illness due to one's behaviour, of course. And that is partly the aim of prophylaxis.

Immunity

Further, homoeoprophylaxis is not an attempt to install some kind of immunity into the body. Natural immunity will, of course, always be assisted by the use of homoeotherapy, though that should not be read as a plea for a homoeoprophylactic programme. However, immunity is neither resistance nor preparedness to *offer* resistance: it is conductivity, and capacity to conduct. Homoeoprophylaxis can never be anything more than an aid to conductivity.

Advance cure

Finally, homoeoprophylaxis is not cure 'in advance'. Simply, one has to become ill before one may be cured. Having said that, one must remember that the intuition of group disease that prompts the patient to request prophylaxis may be thought of as being itself a symptom, in which case the patient's occult illness may be thought of as being bound to respond to the correctly selected prophylactic. And in fact, patients often report an unexpected dispelling of a known, i.e. *current*, problem after taking a prophylactic that was designed for something else.

PRESCRIBING PROTOCOLS

Just as is the case with patients presenting with actual illness, there are various prescribing protocols. In prophylaxis, there are three:

- isopathic
- homoeopathic
- iso-homoeopathic.

The isopathic protocol (isoprophylaxis)

A side effect of the isopathic remedy is to eliminate the specific group disease vector, should it be encountered. That is why we prescribe the vector in potency for the anticipated illness, e.g. Influenzinum 200C for anticipated influenza.

It will also have the effect of weakening the patient's susceptibility to the morphogenetic field influence of the specific group disease, thus affording fractionally increased immunity (which may endure).

Epidemic prophylaxis

Epidemic prophylaxis using nosodes may be achieved using the prescribing programme described in *Group Disease*, below.

In practice, a case of epidemic disease is usually treated on the basis of anticipating clinical therapeutics, first, because the disease is usually well defined, and secondly, because a case that is taken by full repertorisation (e.g. minimising common symptoms) will often give the same result.

Group disease

A patient can be prophylactically assisted to eliminate any group disease influence that is endemic to his environment whether or not a medical epidemic has been declared, e.g. the disease effects of air pollution.

Usually, the group remedy, e.g. the isopathic nosode, would be prescribed when:

- there is a family history of the relevant disease
- there are sequelae to infection and the indicated homoeopathically remedy has failed to ameliorate
- there is a suspected group disease and the homoeopathically indicated remedy has failed to ameliorate
- a prophylactic is required.

The main applications of prophylactic prescribing in homoeopathy occur in relation to childhood disease and in anticipation of the ill-effects of vaccination.

In the absence of an epidemic, the remedial nosode is usually given periodically from an early age, in a potency that will not tax the patient's vital force. The purpose of the introductory course is not to confer immunity, but to prepare the vitalistic terrain for the eventuality of specific illness.

I would add that the introductory course and its maintenance doses are not an attempt to induce a **grafting** of the remedy, in the hope that the organism would thereby achieve a new kind of immune status, for the reasons that, first, grafting always results in an unhelpful state and second, the installation of mechanisms of resistance has nothing to do with vitalistic medicine.

It should be noted that a nosode can always be prescribed homoeopathically when it is the indicated similimum.

Travelling

Patients who are about to travel to areas in which group diseases, e.g. malaria, are endemic, may be prophylactically prepared.

(See also *Homoeopathic protocol: Generic illness*, below.)

Homoeopathic protocol (homoeoprophylaxis)

A prophylactic that is administered *as a similimum* may be prescribed *as if the patient was already* symptomatic. Thus, the practitioner would be required to imagine that the patient was suffering from the illness he wished to mitigate.

This protocol has the advantage that the patient's vital field will already have experienced the installation of a healing gradient (if the symptoms were correctly anticipated), especially if the patient had experienced a proving of the remedy, resulting in a minimising of the disease.

Generic illness

A common use of the similimum for prophylaxis is in the case of anticipated illness while travelling, usually due to food poisoning. Usually, the physician will not be able to anticipate the specific organism that might be encountered by the patient while he is away. However, the patient will be able to voice his concerns, and a compromise simplex (or occasionally, complex) may be prescribed.

Medical procedure

The homoeopathic preparation for an invasive or disturbing medical procedure, i.e. the prophylactic procedure, is to prescribe the remedy that would be prescribed if the patient were to suffer ill-effects of that procedure.

Often, a remedy that has been prescribed as a prophylactic for a medical procedure will continue to be indicated following the procedure.

Ordeal

The homoeopathic preparation for an ordeal: public speaking, dental surgery, etc, is useful, and may be made on the basis of the *Mind, Anticipation* entries in the Repertory.

Iso-homoeopathic protocol (iso-homoeoprophylaxis)

There is nothing to prevent the practitioner from prescribing both isopathics and homoeopathics for the same anticipated illness. The usual rules of prescribing apply, with the special cautions relating to polypharmacy. In this regard, you may wish to review *Polypharmacy*, in Chapter 10, and *Singularity theorem*, in Chapter 12, both in Book 1.

Naturally, modal factors come into play in polypharmacy, especially the presence in the mix of the patient's constitutional (always an amplificational), whether intended or not.

As always, the protocol should be designed to install only the appropriate healing gradient.

I have found it prudent to prescribe both an isopathic and an anticipatory homoeopathic—one of each. The medicines are always dispensed in separate containers, to facilitate dosage control.

VACCINATION

Vaccination is the deliberate introduction into the living organism of a group disease vector, e.g. a microorganism. This has the effect of distressing the organism at all levels, as it lacks the timeliness and vital commensurability appropriate to it.

In that its aim is the disempowerment of the thriving individual, it is not a medical procedure but a political one. Vaccination, being a programme of the subversion and enslavement of the individual, does not occur in vitalistic medicine.

The term *homoeopathic vaccination* is a nonsense. That term, when it is used by non-homoeopaths, may refer to the isopathic treatment of a patient who is about to be vaccinated, in anticipation of vaccination illness, or vaccinosis. The intention in using a homoeopathic as a prophylactic for vaccination would be to minimise the inevitable side–effects of the vaccination.

Also, the term is often loosely (and incorrectly) applied by allopaths to homoeoprophylaxis in anticipation of an epidemic disease, especially one for which an allopathic vaccine has been created. In homoeopathy, neither of those applications is regarded as vaccination.

(See also *Epidemic prophylaxis*, above.)

KEY CONCEPTS

Grafting A response to excessive dosing with a potency, resulting in a patient adopting a permanent compensatory mechanism that may adversely affect behaviour in all spheres.

Homoeopathic prophylaxis (homoeoprophylaxis) A prophylactic prescribing protocol based solely on homoeopathic principles.

Homoeoprophylactic A homoeopathic medicine used as a prophylactic.

Iso-homoeopathic prophylaxis (iso-homoeoprophylaxis) A prophylactic prescribing protocol based the concurrent prescription of homoeopathic and isopathic medicines.

Isopathic prophylaxis (isoprophylaxis) A prophylactic prescribing protocol based solely on the isopathic prescription of group disease vectors in potency.

Isoprophylactic An isopathic medicine used as a prophylactic.

Prophylaxis homoeopathic prescribing in anticipation of a disturbance of the vital force.

Susceptive mode Mode of medicinal action in which remedy acceptability, both immediate and persisting, is enhanced or instilled.

10 - HOMOEOPATHIC PROPHYLAXIS IN PRACTICE

PROPHYLACTIC PROGRAMME
PRESCRIBING PROTOCOLS
Isopathic protocol
Childhood disease and epidemic
International travel
Preparation for vaccination
Homoeopathic protocol
Prior history
No prior history
Cautions
Allopathic medical procedure
Ordeal
Iso-homoeopathic protocol
REMEDY, POTENCY AND DOSAGE
Selecting the appropriate remedy
Selecting the appropriate potency
Dosage
Side effects of prophylaxis

PROPHYLACTIC PROGRAMME

A patient prophylactic programme should be practical and based on sound vitalistic principles. Thus, these medicines should:

- not be given more often than necessary
- cause as little proving as possible
- be designed to achieve a specific effect.

The principle of prophylactic programme design is to install a healing gradient for each specific intended outcome, as there might be a number of concerns. Basically, all that is required to install a healing gradient is a single dose. The rule is: the dose required to install a sufficient healing gradient will be one that matches the patient's current vital force.

The velocity of the required dose will be almost impossible to predict, so the patient should be given fresh exposures at appropriate intervals. A transient aggravation would signal success, though that effect should not be sought.

If the prophylactic is a nosode, a complementary homoeopathic may be dispensed, to be taken later if required.

The most frequently requested programmes involve prophylaxis for:

- international travel
- vaccination
- medical procedures
- childhood disease
- epidemic
- ordeal.

PRESCRIBING PROTOCOLS

In practice, it is customary to prescribe at least one isopathic to eliminate each specific group disease vector, as well as the envisaged similimum. For example, in case of food poisoning, one might prescribe *Salmonella* in potency, together with an appropriate homoeopathic, e.g. (in this case) Veratrum Album.

As described in Chapter 9, three prescribing strategies are available:

- isopathic
- homoeopathic
- iso-homoeopathic.

Isopathic protocol

In the isopathic protocol the practitioner prescribes a specific group disease vector in potency, e.g. Morbillinum in anticipation of contact with measles. Often, polypharmacy is used.

As homoeotherapy is not used in the isopathic protocol (cure not being the aim), the only use for a similimum, in the event of the patient actually become ill as a side effect of detoxification, would be as a palliative, e.g. Nux Vomica for nausea.

Childhood disease and epidemic

When it is not known when the anticipated challenge might strike, the correct course of action is to prescribe a single dose of the nosode immediately, not with the intention of producing a proving, but simply to begin the installation of the healing gradient.

Thus, the typical programme might consist of prescribing the remedy over a brief period, say, three to seven days, immediately prior to the anticipated challenge.

If a proving does occur, then the programme may be regarded as complete, and no further action need be taken unless antidoting is requested. The dose should be repeated at regular intervals, say, every three months, until the danger has passed.

Thus, a typical programme might continue for several years. It is recommended that you begin with a low potency, say, 1LM, and then increase the potency each time the remedy is repeated: 2LM, 3LM, 4LM, etc.

Allopathic drug manufacturers often produce vaccines in response to epidemics. These vaccines may be potentised and used to produce isopathic medicines. However, bear in mind that their other contents: cell culture media, adjuvants, preservatives, and so on, would also be potentised.

International travel

International travellers usually seek prophylaxis in anticipation of extremely dangerous illnesses, e.g. Giardiasis. Polypharmacy is the norm in these cases.

Example Set 10.1 shows the areas in which particular the most common endemic disease have been identified. From time to time, an endemic disease will also be identified in the wake of, for example, a natural disaster.

Example Set 10.1 Prophylactics for international travellers

Ex.	*Region*	*Indication*	*Remedy*
1	Asia	Cholera	Cholerinum
2	Mainly undeveloped countries	Typhoid fever	Typhoidinum
	Mainly undeveloped countries	Paratyphoid fever	Paratyphoidinum
3	Central and South America; tropical Africa	Yellow fever	Yellow Fever Nosode (Aedinum)
4	Africa; South America; Afghanistan	Epidemic typhoid fever	Typhinum

5	Tropics (mainly) and subtropics	Malaria	Malaria Officinalis
6	Africa; Mediterranean zone; Middle East; Central and South America	Leishmaniasis	Leishmaninum
7	South-east Asia; Central America	Plague	Plague Nosode
8	Central America; South-east Asia; India; Tropical coasts	Dengue fever	Dengue Fever Nosode
9	Central and South-east Asia; Pacific Islands	Scrub typhus	Typhinum
10	Africa	African trypanosomiasis (Sleeping sickness)	African Trypanosominum
11	Mainly tropical zones, though worldwide	Giardiasis	Giardinum
12	Africa; Central & South America	American trypanosomiasis (Chagas' disease)	American Trypanosominum
13	Asia	Traveller's diarrhoea[1]	Vibrio Parahaemolyticus Nosode Shigellinum (Dysenterinum) Giardinum Escherichia Coli Nosode Salmonellinum Campylobacter Jejuni Nosode Cholerinum
14	Mainly tropical zones	Amoebiasis	Amoebinum
15	Mainly tropical zones; Africa	Schistosomiasis	Schistosominum

1 The prescriber may decide to prescribe relevant remedies listed in the form of a complex.

Preparation for vaccination

In the following scenario (Example Set 10.2) the situation that is being anticipated is vaccinosis arising out of the administration of pertussis vaccine. In this example, the practitioner would have a much wider range of options than if he were simply prescribing for anticipated whooping cough of what is essentially mysterious aetiology. In this case, there is a clearer aetiology, namely the anticipated vaccination.

Note that, if the patient already had a history of whooping cough-like symptoms following vaccination the vaccination programme would probably not proceed.

Example Set 10.2 Prophylactic options for whooping cough vaccination

Remedy	*Type*	*Mode of application*	*Strategy*
Pertussinum	Nosode	Isopathic	Elimination of *Bordetella pertussis*
Diphtheria Tetanus Pertussis (DTP) Vaccine	Nosode	Isopathic	Elimination of DTP vaccine
DTP Vaccininum	Nosode	Isopathic	Mitigation of anticipated vaccinosis
Pertussis Vaccininum	Nosode	Isopathic	Mitigation of anticipated vaccinosis
Vaccininum	Generic vaccinosis nosode	Isopathic	Vaccinosis

If the patient has already been vaccinated and has become ill as a result, he should first be treated for that illness, even if it appears to have subsided. Such treatment might involve the prescription of a suitable homoeopathic followed by a suitable isopathic.

Having decided to prescribe an isopathic, the prescriber might then decide to concentrate on the vaccine itself, and to prescribe DTP Vaccininum, because the vaccine will be administered as DPT vaccine. Of course, where the patient is already ill and is about to be vaccinated there will be no need to prescribe prophylactically, as vaccination will probably not proceed.

Now, the fact is that it is simply not possible to prevent a disease occurring by the use of a homoeopathic. For example, if one were to prescribe Drosera, one might induce a transient response, i.e. a proving, but its effect would represent the installation of a healing gradient, and the patient would still be free to eventually contract the target group disease, say, whooping cough (though probably not while under the influenced of the homoeopathic).

Homoeopathic protocol

The success of a homoeopathic prophylactic will depend on the healing gradient. Any transient proving that occurs will install lasting susceptibility to the remedy and, logically, neutralises syndromic analogons of itself. However, the absence of a therapeutic proving (due, understandably, to caution) does not mean that the healing gradient is ineffectual, simply that it may be suboptimal.

Naturally, only one medicine should be prescribed as an anticipatory homoeopathic for a given condition—this only applies to proven remedies. They patient may feel more confident if he takes the medicine away with him.

Prior history

Of course, if a certain remedy has worked before, then that will probably be the one selected. Similarly, a patient may have been successfully prescribed a remedy for a similar illness state in the past. Alternately, the patient might have a tendency to display certain symptoms and modalities when ill, owing to the constitutional diathesis.

If a patient has no previous experience of this illness, his homoeopathic history may provide a clue to the remedy. Quite often, a patient will be found to have responded to only a small group of remedies throughout his homoeopathic experience, regardless of his illness presentation. Once that group has been identified, all that remains is to consult the *Materia Medica* to ascertain their suitability.

No prior history

If the patient has no homoeopathic history, or if none of the remedies previously prescribed are suitable, then the *Materia Medica* must be consulted, probably via the Repertory.

Just how far should you carry this envisioning exercise? If the patient is a good observer of his symptoms, you should have no difficulty arriving at the appropriate remedy. Of course, you should always probe a little to discover any invariable general symptoms or modalities the patient is aware of. For example, he might always become hungry and crave strong stimulants when he is ill.

Cautions

When prescribing homoeopathics prophylactically, you should be aware at all times that a potentised remedy can produce a proving in a patient who appears to be healthy, the strength of the proving being proportionate to their susceptibility. This should be explained to the patient.

Also, it is important to remember when prescribing a similimum that it must, as far as possible, be a remedy that would seem to be appropriate for the patient. If a history has been taken for that patient, that should present no problem.

However, if this is the first time you have seen the patient you will need to ask a few questions as to his previous healing response to the type of problem he anticipates. Failing that, a prescription that is at least not incompatible with his general homoeopathic constitution should be considered. A simple solution, given the inadvisability of guessing the proposed remedy, might be to prescribe the patient's constitutional.

The remedies shown in Example Set 10.2 may be prescribed with a nosode simplex or complex, if desired. The only caution with a complex is that the contents should not be homoeopathically incompatible.

Allopathic medical procedure

The homoeopathic preparation for an invasive or disturbing medical procedure, i.e. the prophylactic procedure, is to prescribe the remedy that would be prescribed if the patient were to actually suffer ill effects of that procedure.

Often, a remedy that has been prescribed as a prophylactic for a medical procedure will continue to be indicated following the procedure.

Example Set 10.3 Prophylaxis for medical procedure

Ex.	*Indication*	*Selected example remedies*
1	Cancer chemotherapy	Nux Vomica
2	Catheterisation	Calendula Staphysagria
3	Cautery	Argentum Nitricum Staphysagria
4	Dental extraction	Arnica Hypericum Staphysagria
5	Dental filling	Hypericum Magnesium Phosphoricum Rescue Remedy (Bach)
6	Electroshock therapy	Helleborus Niger Morphinum Phosphorus
7	Eye surgery	Calendula Euphrasia Hypericum Staphysagria
8	Fistula repair	Calendula Silicea
9	Joint surgery	Bryonia
11	Hernia	Hypericum
12	Laparotomy	Opium
13	Lithotomy	Staphysagria
14	Mastectomy	Belladonna Calendula Conium Maculatum
15	Ovariotomy	Staphysagria
16	Wounds	Arnica Bellis Perennis Calendula Hypericum

Ordeal

When prescribing for anticipated ordeal it is usually not necessary to choose from the nosodes. Such remedies may also be used in recovery mode.

Example Set 10.4 Prophylaxis for ordeal

Ex.	*Indication*	*Remedy*
1	Examination anxiety	Gelsemium Sempervirens Mimulus (Bach)
2	Anticipated seasickness	Cocculus Indicus
3	Anticipated traumatic childbirth	Bambusa Vulgaris
4	Anticipated car-sickness	Tabacum

Iso-homoeopathic protocol

In the case of anticipated infectious disease, you might consider it prudent to prescribe both a homoeopathic and an isopathic. It is simply a matter of anticipating the species of challenge, and prescribing the appropriate (isopathic) nosode together with the homoeopathic you consider would work best for that particular patient.

As usual, the single (homoeopathic) remedy caution should be observed. In these cases, the patient may take the isopathic before the anticipated challenge, and the homoeopathic only in the event of actually becoming ill.

REMEDY, POTENCY AND DOSAGE

Selecting the appropriate remedy

The initial assumption in prophylactic prescribing is that the prescriber has precise knowledge of the anticipated illness state.

In Example Set 10.5 the anticipated situation is whooping cough infection, either due to an epidemic or through normal endemic infection. Let us say that the practitioner has decided that the appropriate homoeopathic *for this patient*, would be Drosera. (Note that he might also consider a nosode, to be used isopathically.)

The final choice of a prophylactic will be determined by the extent to which the remedy matches the expected symptoms. If the match is close, it must be because the patient—or perhaps a sibling—has experienced success with the remedy for the disease state in question.

Example Set 10.5 Prophylactic options for whooping cough

Remedy	*Type*	*Mode of application*	*Strategy*
Drosera	Sarcode	Homoeopathic	Mitigation of anticipated illness
Pertussinum	Nosode	Isopathic	1. Elimination of *Bordetella pertussis* 2. Mitigation of anticipated whooping cough

Notes:

1 .For simplicity, we will ignore the possibility of a complex of homoeopathics, though complexes do have their place in 'blind' prophylactic prescribing.
2. Drosera was chosen as an example because it is the most frequently reported curative for pertussis.
3. DTP vaccine in potency would not be considered unless the patient was being treated for the side effects of the vaccine, in which case it would be isotherapeutic.

Other factors that might be taken into consideration in remedy selection include the patient's constitutional, if known, and the clinical specificity of the remedy candidates.

Note that in the absence of reliable indications for a similimum, the remedy would be selected from the available isopathics. In this example, the selected nosode is Pertussinum, for the reason that, given its source, it is more representative of the illness state. (Remember that, in vitalistic medicine *Bordetella pertussis* is not the *cause* of a disease but the *result* of one. Nevertheless, for purely isopathic reasons it could be a viable option, especially if the underlying strategy was simple elimination of the vector.)

Selecting the appropriate potency

Prophylactics are prescribed in low potencies when the prescribing strategy is homoeopathic; and in higher potencies when the strategy is isopathic, i.e. to stimulate specific elimination.

Example Set 10.6 illustrates how prescribing might be carried out. Note that homoeoprophylaxis for an invasive or disturbing medical procedure usually requires prescription of the indicated remedy in low potency, simply because the prescription will be based on common physical symptoms. The exception is where there is a precedent for the prescription *for a particular patient.*

Example Set 10.6 Selection of homoeoprophylactic potencies

Ex.	*Scenario*	*Remedy, potency and dosage*
1	Measles prophylaxis programme	Morbillinum 1M. daily for one week, then every 3 months
2	Anticipated side effects of abdominal surgery	Strontium Carbonicum 6C 3 times a day for 3 days
3	Endoscopy	Silica 20X four times a day for 24 hours.

Dosage

Once the healing gradient has been established, the patient should be instructed to stop taking the remedy, to avoid a proving.

In the vitalistic model there is no need to mimic the periodicity of allopathic vaccination programmes, as the purpose of homoeoprophylaxis is not to build resistance or to sell drugs. Having said that, the practitioner may wish to instruct the patient to take the isopathic periodically, to instil susceptibility.

Side effects of prophylaxis

One of the occasional problems that attends prophylactic prescribing is that of an unexpected proving. If the symptoms are bothersome, the patient might attempt to antidote them homoeopathically, though this will only work on a proving of a homoeopathic, and only if the patient knows how to do it—select a remedy, etc.

If the prophylactic was prescribed isopathically—usually a nosode—that may not be possible, mainly because the remedy will probably be unproven.

Also, the patient may have become ill for an entirely unrelated reason.

APPENDIX
THEORY OF MIASMS

CLASSICAL THEORY
ACUTE VERSUS CHRONIC MIASMS
THE MIASM DECONSTRUCTED
CRITICISM OF THE MIASM THEORY

CLASSICAL THEORY

In classical homoeopathy chronic disease is spoken of as resulting from infection by a *chronic miasm*. It may also include chronic disease caused and be exacerbated by orthodox medical treatment, and industrial and environmental substances. The test of a chronic disease is that, if left to itself, it will get worse, wearing out the vital force.

A chronic miasm is held to be a *taint* that causes the vital force to attempt, unsuccessfully, to be rid of it, causing symptoms. (Acute miasms, also, are attempts by the vital force to be rid of chronic miasms.) Miasms may be inherited, passed on to others, or contracted by contact with noxious substances, e.g. allopathic drugs.

The theory emphasises a protomiasm, known as psora, and numerous derivative miasms, especially the supermiasms: luesis (syphilis), sycosis (gonorrhoea), tuberculosis and cancer. The miasm is typically transmitted via a specific vector, e.g. in the case of the heroin miasm: heroin itself.

ACUTE VERSUS CHRONIC MIASMS

The original three chronic miasms: psora, sycosis and syphilis, were distinguishable from the acute miasms by their characteristic of being permanent and non-fatal. Since then, the definition of the chronic miasm has been widened to include the tubercular, oncotic, malarial and other miasms which are distinguishable from the acute miasms by the fact that their presence does not represent attempts by the vital force to eradicate chronic miasms, as the acute miasms do.

The acute miasms, the acute infectious diseases, are regarded homoeopathically as attempts by the vital force to be rid of (ultimately) psora, the fundamental chronic disease. On this view, the common childhood diseases would be typical miasmic diseases, and their successful passage could be viewed as successful inroads into the fundamental chronic disease.

In fact, it may be readily observed that a suppression of a childhood infectious disease will result in an incompetent immune system and the instatement of chronic disease. The classical nosological observer's interpretation of a given disease picture is that it displays the features of a miasm.

Example Set 1 Types of Miasms

Miasm	*Type*	*Characteristic pathologies*	*Keynote*
Psora	Prototypical supermiasm	Eczematous itch	Underfunction
Luesis	Supermiasm	Chancres and ulcers	Destruction
Sycosis	Supermiasm	Proliferative skin and mucosal changes	Overfunction
Tuberculosis	Supermiasm	Cavitation and exudation	Exhaustion
Cancer	Supermiasm	Tumours	Failure of control
Malaria	Chronic miasm	Fever	Collapse
Vaccination	Chronic miasm	Nervous system disease	Toxicity
Alcoholism	Chronic miasm	Vital organ destruction	Addiction
Rubella	Acute miasm	Rubella	Acuteness

Thus, for example, a tendency to respiratory disorders is often associated with the tubercular miasm, and such a case may be loosely classified as tubercular. The patient may even be prescribed a species of Tuberculinum, e.g. Tuberculinum Bovinum, on the basis that that is the correct way to address the tubercular miasm. That school of thought is strictly isopathic.

The prescriber may then search for a suitable tubercular homoeopathic, e.g. a remedy that both displays a spectrum of 'tubercular' symptoms, e.g. Stannum Metallicum, *and* matches the patient's presentation. In itself, this way of arriving at a remedy may be perfectly valid, despite its bias towards common physical symptoms.

The inescapable fact is that remedies can easily be related to systemic classes of pathology: skin diseases, respiratory disorders, nervous disorders, and so on, and often can be related to specific pathological states, e.g. septicaemia, regardless of miasm theory. What is not so certain is the validity of the theory of miasm as a historical and physical phenomenon.

Naturally, any materialistic theory of disease causation is alien to vitalistic medicine.

THE MIASM DECONSTRUCTED

Given the above information, it should actually be possible to deconstruct a miasm. Why would one want to do so? Because the procedure could have some use, albeit limited, in designing a healing strategy. The procedure used here is that of Koehler[3].

Let us say that an elderly patient presents with an acute disease resembling chickenpox, of which there is a history. The physician recognises the common disease shingles and identifies the causative agent as Herpesvirus IV (varicella zoster virus). We now have the information we need to deconstruct the miasm.

We name the miasm the *chickenpox/shingles miasm* (because it has two common presentations)—and classify it as an acute miasm, because the acuteness of the illness might be helpful during remedy selection and prescription. We identify the group (or common) disease as shingles. This might also be useful in remedy selection, as this particular form of illness is suggestive of a particular group of remedies. The relative nosode, should we decide to prescribe it, will be Varicellinum. The deconstructed

[3] Koehler, Gerhard 1986, *The handbook of homoeopathy: its principles and practice*, trans. A.R. Meuss, Thorsons Publishing Group, Wellingborough, Northamptonshire.

miasm can now be used as the basis for designing the treatment strategy not only for this patient but for other similar patients.

To complete our example, the physician discovers that the remedy for his patient is one commonly given to patients with this disease, say, Rhus Toxicodendron. The remedy works, and the physician decides to eliminate the miasm by prescribing the miasmic: Varicellinum.

Example Set 2 Miasms deconstructed

Miasm	*Type*	*Disease vector &/name of disease*	*Nosode*	*Typical remedy*
Cancer	Chronic	Cancer	Carcinosin	Arsenicum Album
Chickenpox/ Shingles	Acute	Varicella zoster virus Chickenpox/ shingles	Varicellinum	Rhus Toxicoden-dron
Malaria	Chronic	Infected *Anopheles* mosquito[1]	Malaria Officinalis	China Officinalis

1. The vector could also be regarded as any of the species of *Plasmodium* protozoa that cause human malaria. In any case, it is the mosquito that is the carrier.

We can use this process for deconstructing any miasm, then using the result to streamline our decision-making processes. We can also use the model to create an expansive list of typical remedies for each new miasm constructed.

Example Set 2 shows how three miasms may be deconstructed.

CRITICISM OF THE MIASM THEORY

In Book 1 (Chapter 3) we saw that illness left unaddressed flows inevitably into relationships and groups at all levels, and finally into the human specific collective. Healing overtakes this process and neutralises it. The miasm theory, given its physicalist nature, suffers from having been superseded by the microbial and hereditary theories of disease transmission (which it anticipated, though incompletely).

Most homoeopathic physicians would now subscribe to these modern theories, even though they are purely materialistic and suffer from the dubious distinction of having been validated scientifically. For the modern, materialistic homoeopath the shift was a small one. But for the vitalists the original miasmic theory was a backward step.

However, if one were to commit to the idea of the physical causality of disease, then one would have to question the historical explanation of the miasms.

Psora (from Greek psōra 'itch'), and was once considered by homoeopaths to be the primordial human disease. The miasm theory holds that one's earliest attempts at dispelling miasm are the childhood diseases. Now, these are all fevers, and with the exception of chicken pox do not generally overwhelm with their skin symptoms. Could a better explanation of the fundamental disease be devised, while preserving the theory of miasm? Is there a protodisease?

Hahnemann thought of psora as underfunction, but the primary symptomatology in any case of disease is inflammation, which is plainly a series of increases and new activities: fever, pain, malaise, discharge, hyperexcretion, etc. Can we reinstate the miasmic theory by linking it to vitalistic principles?

If we treat miasm as a *group* disease, then we can retain the ideas of noxious influence and mass infection, even of trans-hereditability, but only at the cost of precision. The presumption that the protomiasm was leprosy, for example, was simply a guess. Do we all have leprosy, as we all 'have' the protomiasm psora? It is pointless to go on wondering. In any case, it is a gross oversimplification to refer to leprosy as a skin disease. Thus the credibility gap widens.

Thus, also, the homoeopathic theory of the natural evolution of leprosy into sexually transmitted disease, as represented by the evolution of psora into sycosis and syphilis, may also be considered dubious.

Group disease theory is posited as a new way of thinking about and treating disease using homoeopathic medicines.

KEY CONCEPTS

Acute miasm In miasm theory, an acute miasm is an acute infectious disease which the organism gets in order to be rid of a chronic miasm.

Chronic miasm In miasm theory, a taint that permanently but not fatally disturbs the vital force. It may be inherited or contracted by contact with miasmic material.

Nosode A medicine prepared from a pathological product. Nosodes are used in the treatment of group disease.

Supermiasm Any of the greater miasms of miasm theory, especially those that are deemed to be stem miasms: psora, sycosis, luesis.

SERIES GLOSSARY

A

Actual medical power The product of a remedy's intrinsic curative power and its nominal numerical potency.

Acute disease A disease that is self-limiting, i.e. ending in recovery or death, and is frankly symptomatic. *See also* **chronic disease; pseudo-chronic disease**.

Acute miasm In **miasm theory**, an acute miasm is an acute infectious disease which the vital force contracts in order to be rid of a chronic miasm. *See also* **group disease**.

Aetiology Causation.

Aggravation **1. Allopathic a.** Iatrogenic poisoning. **2. Homoeopathic a.** An acute transient episode of the presenting symptoms following homoeopathic medication. It is due to an apparent acceleration of the life force in the direction of the desuppression. **3. Isopathic a.** An aggravation of symptoms following the administration of an isopathic medicine. It is due to a proving of the **vector**. **4. Constitutional a.** Transient symptomatic amplification following administration of the **constitutional**.

Allopathic aggravation *See* **aggravation (1)**.

Alternating remedies Remedies that tend to appear in alternation in the course of a case.

Amelioration Improvement. The lifting of suppression.

Ameliorative mode of medicinal response The patient exhibits complete or limited improvement. Seen in **cure, palliation, constitutional improvement, prophylaxis, and antidoting**.

Amplificational mode Mode of medicinal action in which the patient exhibits an increase in vitality (resulting in aggravation, if symptomatology exists), often seen after the constitutional is administered. *See* also: **curative m., eliminative m., palliative m., probative m., restorative m., supportive m.,** and **susceptive m.**

Amplifier A remedy that amplifies the symptom picture.

Analogue-icon A symbolic representation of a remedy which may be used to produce a medicine.

Analogy theorem A disturbance of the vital force will be annihilated by a remedy that is sufficiently reminiscent of (i.e. specifically analogous to) its abnormal organismic expression.

Anamnesis *See* **case taking.**

Annihilation (of disturbance-resistance complex) Healing. In particular, the resolution of symptoms by the presentation of a specific symptom analogue.

Anthroposophical medicine A branch of vitalistic medicine in which potentialised medicines are prescribed using anthroposophical principles.

Antidote A remedy that has been selected for the purpose of neutralising the ill-effects of a remedy which has been incorrectly prescribed.

Antidoted by A subheading of *Relations* given in a remedy's entry in the *Materia Medica*, which gives its occasional antidotes. *See* **antidote.**

Antidotes to A subheading of *Relations* given in a remedy's entry in the *Materia Medica*, which mentions remedies it occasionally antidotes. *See* **antidote.**

Antipathic Of antipathy, i.e. therapy designed to suppress the vital force.

Ascending collective dose A form of **collective dose** in which the potency is fractionally increased before each administration.

Autopathic A potentialised medicine made from the patient himself, hence **autopathy**.
Autopathy *See* **autopathic**.

C

Case taking Anamnesis. The process of discovering the patient's presenting problem and it symptoms, what is to be cured, and the depth of disturbance of the patient's vital energy. Together these discoveries constitute the **totality of the case**.
Centesimal scale A standard scale of potency, on which successive potencies are deconcentrated in the ratio 1:100. *See also* **deconcentration; scale of potency**.
Central disturbance The disturbance that has triggered the presentation. *See also* **disturbance**.
Characteristic symptoms The symptoms that are most characteristic of a remedy.
Chronic disease A cycle of similar acute illnesses with a constant background of pain, dysfunction or immobility at any or all levels of eccentricity. *See also* **acute disease; pseudo-chronic disease**.
Chronic miasm In **miasm theory**, a taint that permanently but not fatally disturbs the vital force. It may be inherited or contracted by contact with miasmic material. *See also* **group disease**.
Chronicity 1. The time elapsed since the onset of symptoms. **2. C of symptoms**. A result of the failure of the life force to complete its timely expression through the organism.
Clinical application Legitimate clinical use for a potentialised medicine. These are: constitutional therapy, isopathy, cure, palliation, prophylaxis.

Clinical diagnosis The allocation of a syndrome to a pathophysiological family.

Clinical remedies In **clinical therapeutics**, remedies that are often indicated for diagnosed diseases.

Collaterals Remedies that resemble each other by virtue of their source substances belonging to the same family, e.g. a plant family or a column of the Periodic Table. *See also* **compatibles; family resemblance**.

Collective dose A dose of a given potentialised medicine, when dispensed as a set of exposures.

Comparable A remedy that strongly resembles a given remedy in at least one area of symptomatology. *See also* **compatibles**.

Compatibles A class of remedies that have similar leading symptoms, and are at least not mutually *in*compatible. Compatibles include **collaterals**, **comparables**, **complementaries**, remedies that **follow well**, and remedies that are **followed well (by)**. *See also* **incompatibles**.

Complementaries A class of remedies that is said to complete the action of the similimum when there are residual symptoms. *See also* **compatibles**.

Complete symptom A symptom that has been described in terms of its time, location, sensation, intensity, modality and **concomitant symptoms**, if there are any.

Complicated case A case that has a complex of aetiologies.

Concomitant symptoms Symptoms that occur simultaneously and do not seem to have any logical relationship.

Concurrent medication The prescribing of two or more remedies without waiting for the action of each remedy to be exhausted.

Concurrent remedies Remedies whose courses of action at least partly coincide. *See* **concurrent medication**.

Constitution The complete organism in all of its spheres: behavioural, intellectual, emotional, physical, being the sum of all that it has inherited and acquired. *See also* **constitutional; constitutional diathesis; constitutional prescribing; constitutional remedy**.

Constitutional aggravation Transient symptomatic amplification following administration of the **constitutional**.

Constitutional diathesis The features of a given constitution that leads it to be susceptible to specific morbific agents or influences and predisposed to specific forms of illness.

Constitutional prescribing Prescribing a remedy that matches the patient's apparent constitutional picture, for the purpose of amplifying the patient's vital force.

Constitutional, -al remedy A remedy that is reminiscent of the constitution of a patient.

Curative action The action of a medicine as the result of its resemblance to the presenting symptoms.

Curative mode A mode of medicinal action in which the similimum acts. *See also*: **amplificational mode., eliminative m., palliative m., probative m., restorative m., supportive m.,** and **susceptive m**.

Curative species analogue **1.** The essence that most resembles a given disturbance-resistance complex in its symptomatogenicity. **2.** In homoeopathy, the similimum.

Cure The complete removal of an illness state, including the removal of the primary disturbance-resistance complex.

D

Decimal scale A standard **scale of potency**, on which successive potencies are deconcentrated in the ratio 1:10. *See also* **deconcentration; scale of potency**.

Deconcentration **1.** A **potency** whose creation has involved placing a small quantity of a **mother tincture** (or **mother power**) into a larger quantity of a ritually used substance, usually water. **2.** This process (classical: *dilution*). *See also* **potentialisation**.

Degree of chronicity The time elapsed since the highest degree of symptoms first appeared.

Detoxication *See* **detoxification**.

Detoxification Drainage. The elimination from the organism of toxins that have become obstacles to cure, using potentised remedies, especially isopathically. It includes the elimination of any toxins that it is within the power of the medicine to remove, where a toxin is defined as anything physical or non-physical that naturally causes the vital force to become distorted or stalled.

Detoxification combination A combination of (usually two) medicines used in a detoxification strategy, consisting of: an ***initiator or elimination remedy*** (the remedy prescribed in the higher potency) and a ***support (or protective remedy*** (the remedy prescribed in the lower potency). These **concurrent remedies** are prescribed as two separate simplexes, giving control over the adjustment of dosage.

Detoxification strategy A plan for detoxifying a patient, typically involving the prescription of a **detoxification combination** together with appropriate supporting measures, e.g. lifestyle adjustment.

Diathesis *See* **constitutional diathesis**.

Dilution 1. A mother tincture, usually in the form of a tincture or solution, typically of a poisonous material. **2.** The process of **deconcentration**. *See also* **potentialisation**.

Dimension of illness A factor in the form of a disease presentation. An illness has dimensions of scale, location, symptomatology, spectrum, intensity, chronicity, phase and depth.

Dimension of potency A factor in the power of a potentialised medicine. A homoeopathic medicine has the dimensions of frequency (equivalent to attenuation), phase (equivalent to the force achieved by succession), scale (of attenuation, equivalent to sphere of action), and velocity (of dosage, achieved by repetition). *See also* **scale of potency**.

Direct elimination 1. Elimination that is achieved by the use of isotherapy and homoeotherapy together. **2.** Detoxification, when used as a deliberate strategy.

Disease polarity The manifestation of disease as an opposition of tensions: (inner) pathophysiology and (outer) its solution.

Disordered case A case in which inappropriate homoeopathic prescribing has occurred.

Disturbance Disturbance of the life force. Resistance. It is disturbance of the life force that causes the organism to become diseased.

Disturbance-resistance complex The blockage of the vital force that is the essence of a health problem.

Divided dose dispensing The extempore dispensing, often by a carer, of a **collective dose** at an experimental low potency, to induce initial susceptibility while controlling aggravation. Typically, this kind of dosing would be performed often, and by sipping from a glass, with succussion by stirring.

Dosage The amount of exposure to a medicine.

Dose A single exposure or collection of exposures to a given potentialised medicine.
Drainage *See* **detoxification.**

E

Elimination response An increase in the elimination of toxins, often accompanied by symptoms.
Eliminative mode Mode of medicinal action in which the patient exhibits increased mental and emotional activity, with physiological elimination. The primary mode of **isopathy**. *See also*: **amplificational mode., curative m, palliative m., probative m., restorative m, supportive m.,** and **susceptive m.**
Emotional sphere The sphere of emotional disturbance.
Empathic neutralisation The automatic neutralisation by the similimum of a physician's own empathic 'proving' of the patient. It protects the physician from the accumulated effects of 'burn-out'.
Empathic symptom A symptoms of the patient that are experienced by the physician. *See also* **transference; medical intuition.**
Endotoxin Endogenous toxin. Substance or influence that is generated by the organism in response to disturbance. Endotoxins include mental and physical pathological products. Compare **exotoxin.**
Entelechy An organism's governing intelligence.
Epidemic prescribing Prescribing with a view to eliminating a group disease. It is facilitated by the association of certain remedies with group syndromes (especially in the case of the infectious diseases) that are all manifestations of group syndromes and have their own associated remedies.

Esoteric medicine The division of medicine that deals with the vital force. Its branches include: Qi gong, pranic healing, psychic healing, reflexology, homoeopathy, and psychotherapy.
Essence 1. A remedy; a potential medicine. **2.** One of the forms of mother tincture made by exposing the whole creature to water, alcohol or glycerine. **3. E.** of the disturbance: the nature of the disturbance.
Euthenic, euthenic therapy In **obstetric homoeopathy**, the use of an isopathics to remove the influence of a group disease from the mother.
Exogenous disease A disease that is regarded as having resulted from the ingestion of an exogenous toxin.
Exotoxin Exogenous toxin. A substance or influence that has been drawn into the organism in response to disturbance. Compare **endotoxin**.
Expansive A remedy that amplifies the symptom picture by throwing the **diathesis** into relief.
Extended divided dose dispensing **Divided dose dispensing** with the additional dimension of deconcentration, done by placing a drop of the medicine in a fresh glass of water, before stirring and dispensing.
External sphere The sphere of life in which the patient lives, comprising relationship, resources and environment.

F

Family of remedies A group of remedies having a common set of distinctive symptoms. *See* **family resemblance; remedy relationship**.
Family resemblance A set of symptoms suggesting a group of remedies, and thereby classified as a family. *See* **remedy relationship**.

Feedback mechanism The evaluative mechanism of an organism's governing intelligence during healing.
Final dilution The dilution of a **mother tincture**, usually 1:10.
Followed well (by), is Said of a remedy that has reputed sequels.
Follows well Said of a remedy reputed to be the indicated second or sequel remedy for any fresh symptom picture that appears after the previous total symptom picture has completely resolved homoeopathically. *See also* **compatibles**.
Frequency When applied to **potency**, it is one of dimensions of a vitalistic medicine, expressed as attenuation. In homoeopathic pharmacy it is traditionally (but not necessarily) produced by serial dilution or deconcentration, giving rise to 'potencies', e.g. the 60th potency.
Fundamental postulate of the vitalistic hypothesis Life has a kind of force, being eternal, pure, intelligent, radiant, integral, limitless, independent, thriving, fluid, implicate and apparent, which expresses and explicates itself in the dimensions of growth, proliferation, diversity and beauty; and which manifests as apparent crystalline event-forms.

G

Gemmotherapy The use of low potency (Ø & 1D) phytotherapeutics manufactured from buds and prescribed on clinical indications alone, as agents of detoxification.
General symptom A symptom involving the whole patient.
Genetic scale. The scale of the patient's and the patient's family, racial group or species.
Grafting A response to excessive dosing with a potency, resulting in a patient adopting a permanent compensatory mechanism that may adversely affect behaviour in all spheres.

Group disease A disease of a group. It corresponds, by a factor of scale, to an individual disease. *See* **miasm theory**.
Group disease remedy A signature remedy which is evoked by the diseased group from nature (the externality to which it aspires), and which belongs to the family of isopathics.
Group disease vector A communicable noxious influence whose establishment in the individual signals acceptance of disease.
Group syndrome The symptomatology of a **group disease**.
Growth through illness model To the extent that the patient is in a state of health, he will experience a useful evaluative state, and the feedback to its controlling intelligence will assist it in finding a new centre from which to thrive.

H

Healing characteristics theorem Radiant healing occurs with the characteristics of the life force.
Healing gradient **1.** The natural inclination of the organism to heal. **2.** The inclination to heal that is installed when a potentialised medicine is administered.
Healing motion theorem Healing, once begun, will proceed automatically as a reflection of the qualities of the vital force.
Healing Partnership An agreement by a physician and a patient to do whatever they can to bring about amelioration. The establishment and continuation of a healing partnership is a precondition for cure.
Healing potential theorem The potential of the life force to heal itself will be indicated by the dramatic quality of the symptoms.
Healing rule Essences exert healing power in proportion as their administration is reminiscent of syndromes.

Healing tension The motive force behind healing, which, assists in the resolution of the aetiology-currency tension. In homoeopathic medicine, it is imparted by the dose.
Health A state of freedom of expression of the organism.
Hierarchy of symptoms The ranking order of the main classes of symptoms. The order reflects the spheres of eccentricity of the life force that have been deduced from patient observations. The five classes of symptoms, in descending order of importance are: behavioural, intellectual, emotional, general physical or generalised sensations, particular or localised physical.
Holonomic signature theorem Each species signifies its potential medical use in a unique way by pointing, more or less clearly, to a corresponding set of anatomical, physiological and pathophysiological relationships in every other species.
Homoeopathic *See* **homoeopathic medicine.**
Homoeopathic aggravation *See* **aggravation (2).**
Homoeopathic detoxification *See* **detoxification.**
Homoeopathic Materia Medica *See* **materia medica.**
Homoeopathic medicine **1.** A branch of **vitalistic medicine** in which cure is achieved by medication with potentialised **essential species analogues** of the presenting syndrome. **2.** A remedy when prescribed as the similimum.
Homoeopathic prophylaxis (homoeoprophylaxis) A prophylactic prescribing protocol based solely on homoeopathic principles.
Homoeopathy *See* **homoeopathic medicine.**
Homoeoprophylactic A homoeopathic medicine used as a prophylactic.
Homoeoprophylaxis *See* **homoeopathic prophylaxis.**
Hormonotherapy A branch of **organotherapy** using potentised endocrine products.

Hyposensitisation Isopathic treatment designed to desensitise patients to substances.

I

Idiosyncratic symptom A symptom that is peculiar to an individual.

Illness polarity The simultaneous manifestation of an illness and the essential possibility of its resolution.

Incomparable A remedy that does not resemble a primary remedy candidate in its major symptoms, and may therefore be rejected as a remedy candidate.

Incurable illness **1.** In homoeopathic medicine, disease in which the dominant aetiology-symptomatology complex cannot be resolved, usually because of an obstacle to the curative routine. **2.** Disease in which there has been virtual destruction of a vital organ.

Indirect elimination The elimination of toxins which is routinely achieved as a by-product of homoeotherapy. Compare **direct elimination**.

Inimical A remedy that has been observed to follow a specific remedy with unsatisfactory results, i.e. spoiling the effect of their antecedent, and which therefore have a poor reputation as a sequel.

Initiator remedy In a detoxification combination, the remedy prescribed in the higher potency, usually an isopathic designed to initiate and maintain elimination of a group disease vector. Compare with **support remedy**.

Integration **1.** The resolution of the disease polarity by the mutual annihilation of a vital disturbance and a homoeopathic medicine. **2.** A healing shift felt by the patient. Compare **avoidance**.

Intention The state of awareness of the homoeopathic physician that causes healing to occur. A principle of **case taking**.

Intercurrent remedy A remedy prescribed for an apparently unrelated acute symptom picture that appears during treatment of a chronic disease.

Iso-homoeopathic prophylaxis (iso-homoeoprophylaxis) A prophylactic prescribing protocol based the concurrent prescription of homoeopathic and isopathic medicines.

Isopathic Of a medicine, being made from the same species that caused the disease.

Isopathic aggravation *See* **aggravation (3)**.

Isopathic prescribing The prescribing of a homoeopathic medicine on the principle that a specific and not generic (i.e. similar) match will result in the annihilation of a form of resistance that is identifiable with a group disease. Isopathics are often prescribed for the elimination of group disease **morphogenetic fields**, and with them, group disease vectors, leading to partial or specific detoxification of the individual.

Isopathic prophylaxis (isoprophylaxis) A prophylactic prescribing protocol based solely on the isopathic prescription of group disease vectors in potency.

Isopathy Treatment of group disease by administering a potentised group disease vector.

Isoprophylactic An isopathic medicine used as a prophylactic.

Isoprophylaxis *See* **isopathic prophylaxis**.

L

Law of homoeopathic efficacy The closer the analogy of the symptomatogenicity of the remedy is to the symptomatology of the illness, the more effective the medicine will be. A corollary of the **analogy theorem**.

Law of similars *See* **analogy theorem.**
Law of the minimum dose See **minimality theorem.**
Law of the single dose *See* **posoequivalence theorem.**
Law of the single remedy *See* **singularity theorem.**
LM scale The 50-millesimal scale.

M

Maintaining cause The sustaining factor in a case of **pseudo-chronic disease.**
Materia medica 1. The contents of the homoeopathic pharmacy. **2.** ***Homoeopathic Materia Medica*** The published summaries of provings and related information.
Mediation of medicine The process by which the vitalistic physician transmits the patient's medicine, consisting of a series of steps commencing with case taking, and ending with the presencing of the medicine.
Medical force indicating device (MFID) Expression of magnitude of a remedy's medical force, e.g. Lycopodium 200C.
Medical intuition Knowledge of a patient, and, therefore, of the remedy, obtained by empathic resonance.
Medicinal substance A part of the world whose essence is valued for its intrinsic healing potential, and may be transformed into a medicine.
Medicine 1. The technology of healing. **2.** In homoeopathy, a remedy that has been potentised for a particular patient.
Metaremedy A remedy discovered by the physician after observing his own empathic proving of the patient. It may be used to elicit a clearer symptom picture.
Miasmic A remedy that is strongly associated with a specific miasm, e.g. Nitricum Acidum; Syphilinum (luetic miasm).

Minimality theorem A disturbance of the life force will be annihilated by precisely the quantum of medicine that will cause the life force to resume its expression of the disturbance.

Minimum dose *See* **minimality theorem**.

Minimum potency *See* **minimality theorem**.

Modality **1.** An ameliorating or aggravating factor. **2.** A therapeutic approach. **3.** A remedial display of modal dynamics, e.g. cure.

Modes of medicinal response There are eight: amplificational, curative, eliminative, palliative, probative, restorative, supportive, and susceptive. (See each, separately.)

Morbific agent or influence Whatever will disturb the **vital force**.

Morphic field Resonant field. See also **morphogenetic field**.

Morphic resonance Harmonic attunement resulting in reverberative propagation, and synchronisation.

Morphogenetic field A self-organising and self-remembering, spatio-temporal, vibratory, pattern-imposing, probabilistic field shared by co-resonating members.

Mother power The first potency on a given scale, which is used to create all higher potencies.

Mother tincture Symbol Ø. The form given to the original sample of the remedy species, usually manufactured destructively, in order that medicines can conveniently be manufactured. The most common forms of mother tinctures are: essence, tincture, solution, and trituration.

N

Nosode A remedy prepared from a pathological product. Compare **sarcode**

O

Obstacle to cure Any factor that impedes cure.

Order of cure In the holistic medical strategy the order is: first, the removal of obstacles to cure; second, detoxification; third, homoeotherapy as indicated by the symptomatology most in evidence or emphasised, including aetiology.

Order of healing theorem As healing progresses pathology retrogresses.

Organic sphere The sphere of physical particular symptoms, where the range of remedies that suggest themselves is very wide.

Organotherapy Non-homoeopathic treatment which allegedly facilitates development of specific organs.

P

Paediatric homoeopathy The branch of homoeopathic medicine that deals with symptomatology associated with childhood.

Palliation The use of homoeopathic medicines to relieve suffering, without the expectation of cure.

Palliative mode A mode of medicinal action designed to bring about rapid relief. *See also*: **amplificational m., curative m., eliminative m., probative m., restorative m., supportive m.,** and **susceptive m.**

Pathognomonic symptom A symptom commonly associated with a pathological diagnosis.

Patient The presenter of symptoms.

Pharmacological data Data obtained from toxicological and pharmacological tests of crude substances, accidental poisonings, tests on animals, homoeopathic provings, observations of hospital patients, intuitive discoveries, feedback from patients, and reports of environmental and industrial poisonings.

Pharmacological uniqueness theorem Each pharmacological source is unique in its actions, curative powers and manifestations.

Pharmakon In the medical domain of vitalistic pharmacy, the outer aspect of a disease polarity in the form of its signature solution; in homoeopathy, known as a remedy.

Phase Of a potency, its power, expressed, in classical mechanistic pharmacy, as the number of succussions per deconcentration on a given scale.

Plussing The practice of succussing a medicine before it is dispensed, usually by succussing the medicine bottle 5-10 times, for the purpose of increasing its potency.

Polarity A simultaneous manifestation of an illness and the essential possibility of its resolution.

Polychrest A remedy having a wide spectrum of symptoms.

Posoequivalence theorem A single disturbance of the life force will call for a single dose of the medicine that will initiate cure.

Posology The study of dosage. In homoeopathy it is concerned solely with the measure of the patient's exposure to the remedy.

Potency **1.** Curative power. **2.** Magnitude of curative power expressed as a **medical force indicating device (MFID)**.

Potency selection The creation of a potency that will match the patient's resistance to the flow of the vital force, thereby annihilating it.

Potentialisation A process by which the essential healing nature of a remedy is transformed into a curative power or esoteric medicine.

Potentialised (Of a medicine) curatively enhanced or activated.

Potentisation The initial pharmaceutical process of serial deconcentration and succussion of a sacrificially prepared essence, usually for the purpose of carrying out an experimental proving or preparing off-shelf-potencies.

Preconditions for cure They are: healing partnership, remedy similarity, simplicity, potentiality, and sufficiency.

Primary response The initial response to an influence, e.g. the administration of a potency. Typically the organism experiences stimulation. *See also* **grafting; secondary response; tertiary response**.

Probative mode Mode of medicinal action in which a proving of the remedy occurs. *See also*: **amplificational m., curative m., eliminative m., restorative m., supportive m.,** and **susceptive m**.

Procurative state A state through which an organism passes during its healing response. The procurative states are: organismic behaviour, emotion, organic behaviour, sensation, and extraorganismic events.

Prophylactic proving A **proving** occasionally seen in a patient who has taken a remedy as a prophylactic, especially if he has not exercised caution in self-dosing.

Prophylaxis Homoeopathic prescribing in anticipation of a disturbance of the vital force.

Propositions of homoeopathy The set of theorems that provide the guides and rationalisation for homoeopathic medicine.

Proving **1.** The experimental process of discovering an essence's intrinsic curative powers by medication with the essence in potency. **2.** Unintended or accidental manifestation of a remedy's symptom picture following clinical medication. *See also* **prophylactic proving**.

Pseudo-chronic disease A category of disease that resembles chronic disease but always is sustained by repeated exposures to a morbific agent.

Q

Quinquagintamillesimal scale The 50-millesimal or 1:50,000 **scale of potency**. Abbr. LM or Q.

R

Rapport A state of low resistance to the patient, resulting in the sharing of knowledge at all levels, and facilitating all aspects of case taking. *See also* **preconditions for cure; transference**.

Relevate Raise a potentially curative substance to medical relevance as a **pharmakon**.

Remedy A potential solution to a medical problem. *See* **essence**.

Remedy cycle A recurrent remedy series.

Remedy diagnosis Drug diagnosis. The deduction of the appropriate remedy.

Remedy relationship The alleged homoeopathic relations between remedies. These relations (which appear as supplements to *Materia Medica* entries) have been classified according to their practical usefulness, and are: ***antidotes*** **by**, **antidotes to**, ***comparables***, ***compatibles***, ***inimicals***, ***complementaries***, and ***incompatibles***. *See* **family resemblance**.

Remedy series A series of three or more compatible remedies that have frequently been observed.

Repertory The separately published index to the ***Homoeopathic Materia Medica***.

Resistance In medicine, the preventing factor in dysfunctional disturbance expression.

Restorative mode Mode of medicinal action following homoeotherapy in which the patient's post-curative life changes for the better. *See also*: **amplificational m., curative m., eliminative m., probative m., supportive m.,** and **susceptive m.**

Rule of suppression Symptoms are transformed harmfully as they are artificially turned inwards and concentrated on more internal structures.

S

Sacrificial annihilation The annexation of a specific part of the world and liberation of its essence in order to manufacture a medicine.

Sarcode A medicine prepared from a healthy biological whole creature, or its tissues, secretions or excretions. Compare **nosode**.

Second prescription Any prescription which follows the initial homoeopathic prescription.

Secondary response The second-stage response of an organism to an influence, e.g. the administration of a potency. Typically the organism experiences acute pathology accompanied by increased elimination. *See also* **grafting; primary response; tertiary response**.

Similarity requirement *See* **analogy theorem**.

Similimum The essential curative species analogue of a disease presentation.

Single dose *See* **posoequivalence theorem**.

Single remedy *See* **singularity theorem**.

Singularity theorem The exquisite degree of idiosyncrasy that characterises a singular disturbance will call for a singular remedy. In classical parlance, this is known as the law of the single remedy.

Species analogue Similimum. An essence that resembles a given disturbance-resistance complex in its symptomatogenicity.

Specific A remedy (usually one of several) that is indicated by a clinical diagnosis. *See also* **clinical therapeutics; epidemic remedy**.

Sphere of vitality Any of the spheres of expression of the vital force: organismic behaviour; emotion; organic behaviour; sensation; external world.
Split dose A dose of a homoeopathic medicine that anticipates an interruption, e.g. sleep. It is given before and after the interruption.
Succussion A stage of **potentisation**, consisting of imparting serial shocks to a solution to 'potentise' or 'dynamise' it. The effect is to set the phase of the potency. *See* **phase of potency**.
Supermiasm Any of the greater miasms of miasm theory, especially those that are deemed to be stem miasms: psora, sycosis, luesis.
Support remedy In a detoxification combination, the remedy prescribed in the lower potency, usually for the support and protection of organs of elimination. Compare with **initiator remedy**.
Supportive mode Mode of medicinal action in which the role of the medicine is the support of an organ or system, especially during detoxification. *See also*: **amplificational m., curative m., eliminative m., probative m., restorative m.,** and **susceptive m.**
Suppressive medication Medicine that is prescribed antipathically, i.e. for the purpose of preventing symptoms.
Susceptibility The ability to be infected by a given group influence or vector, including a known remedy. Clinically, susceptibility may be instilled, enhanced or made permanent.
Susceptive mode Mode of medicinal action in which remedy acceptability, both immediate and persisting, is enhanced or instilled. *See also*: **amplificational m., curative m., eliminative m., probative m., restorative m.,** and **supportive m.**
Symptom A datum elicited from the patient concerning illness. Symptoms include: complaints; clinical signs; the results of

laboratory pathology tests; observations, including the observations of witnesses.

Symptomatogenicity The power of a potentised essence to elicit symptoms.

Symptomatogenicity theorem The **curative powers** of a specific manifestation of the life force can be partially ascertained by medicating a relatively asymptomatic individual with it.

T

Terminal illness An illness that will end with the death of the patient. It is therefore a kind of incurable illness.

Tertiary response The third and final stage of response to an influence, e.g. the administration of a potency. Typically the organism experiences a sacrificial or destructive mode, having been forced to find a way of adapting to overwhelm. *See also* **grafting; primary response; secondary response**.

Tincture In pharmacy, the result of extracting the parts of a creature by maceration or percolation in water, alcohol or glycerine.

Total symptom picture The totality of symptoms. The set of symptoms on which the homoeopathic prescription is based.

Totality of symptoms *See* **total symptom picture**.

Totality of the case The totality of the case comprises the patient's presenting problem and it symptoms, what is to be cured, and the dimensions of the disturbance of the patient's vital energy.

Transference Inoculation of the physician with the patient's disease state, a phenomenon that is automatic during rapport.

Transformation Potentialisation. The process of converting essence into medicine.

Treatment strategy A plan for individual treatment, counselling, review, treatment support and patient advice.

V

Vaccination Mass biosuppression. In allopathic medicine, the mass administration of toxic doses of biological **group disease vectors**, called vaccines, with the intention of suppressing symptoms. *See* **mass suppression; also mass chemosuppression.**
Vaccinosis The generic group disease caused by **vaccination**.
Vector *See* **group disease vector**.
Vital force The life force. That which expresses itself in the world. *See* **vitalistic hypothesis.**
Vitalistic hypothesis *See* **fundamental postulate of the vitalistic hypothesis**.
Vitalistic medicine **1.** The division of medicine concerned with the expression of the life force. **2.** A potentialised medicine.
Vitalistic physician One who uses a *medical* technology to mediate and presence medicines in order to facilitate the annihilation of **disturbance-resistance complexes** of the vital force.
Vitoequivalence theorem The power of a curative stimulus is commensurate with the potential of the life force to express in a timely manner the sphere in which it has stalled.
Vortexing Ritual stirring done for the purpose of raising the increasing the phase of a potency. *See* **Phase of potency.**

SERIES BIBLIOGRAPHY & FURTHER READING

Anthropsophical medicine

Bott, Victor 1984, *Anthroposophical medicine: spiritual science and the art of healing,* Healing Arts Press, Rochester, Vermont.

Evans, Michael and Rodger, Iain 1992, *Anthroposophical medicine: treating body, soul and spirit,* Thorsons, Hammersmith.

Husemann, F. and Wolff, O. (eds) 1987, *The anthroposophical approach to medicine: an outline of a spiritual scientifically oriented medicine,* 3 vols, Anthroposophic Press, Bell's Pond, Hudson, NY.

King, Francis X. 1987, *Rudolph Steiner and holistic medicine,* Nicolas-Hays, Inc, York Beach, Maine.

Steiner, Rudolph and Wegman, Ita 1983, *Fundamentals of therapy: an extension of the art of healing through spiritual knowledge,* 4th edn, trans. E.A. Frommer and J.M. Josephson, Rudolph Steiner Press, London.

Case taking

Dhawale, M L 1985, *Principles and practice of homoeopathy,* 2nd edn, Institute of Clinical Research, Bombay.

Gray, Alastair C. 2011, *The landscape of homeopathic medicine,* 3 vols, B. Jain Archibel, Assesse, Belgium.

Koehler, Gerhard 1986, *The handbook of homeopathy: its principles and practice,* trans. A.R. Meuss, Thorsons Publishing Group, Wellingborough, Northamptonshire.

Nash, E.B. n.d., *How to take a case,* B. Jain Publishers, New Delhi.

Patel, R.P. 1990, *The art of practical case taking and practical repertorisation in homoeopathy,* 5th edn, Sai Homoeopathic Book Corporation, Kottayam.

Rowe, Todd 1998, *Homoeopathic methodology: repertory, case taking and analysis,* North Atlantic Books, Berkeley, California.

Roy, Margaret 1994, *The principles of homoeopathic philosophy,* Churchill Livingstone, Edinburgh.

Vithoulkas, George 1980, *The science of homeopathy,* B. Jain Publishers, New Delhi.

Constitution

Beenadas, Dr Apr, 2012, *Role of constitution in homeopathy,* <https://www.homeobook.com/role-of-constitution-in-homeopathy/>

Borland, Douglass M. n.d., *Children's types,* B. Jain Publishers, New Delhi.

Coulter, Catherine R. 1986, *Portraits of homoeopathic medicines: psychophysical analyses of selected constitutional types,* North Atlantic Books, Berkeley, California.

Gaier, Harald C. 1991, *Thorsons encyclopaedic dictionary of homoeopathy: the definitive reference to all aspects of homoeopathy,* Thorsons, Hammersmith, London.

Gray, Alastair C. 2011, *The landscape of homeopathic medicine,* 3 vols, B. Jain Archibel, Assesse, Belgium.

Herscu, Paul 1991, *The homeopathic treatment of children: paediatric constitutional types,* North Atlantic Books, Berkeley, California.

Howard, Wendy April, 2013, *Philosophical constitution,* <https://hpathy.com/homoeopathy-papers/>.

Jefferies, Helen, Welch, Elle & Santiago, Paloma Vazquez Jul, 2013, *Susceptibility,* <https://hpathy.com/organon-philosophy/susceptibility-2/>

Kent, James Tyler n.d., *Lectures on homeopathic philosophy, reprint,* B. Jain Publishers, New Delhi.

Koehler, Gerhard 1986, *The handbook of homeopathy: its principles and practice,* trans. A.R. Meuss, Thorsons Publishing Group, Wellingborough, Northamptonshire.

Poole, Jennifer Apr, 2016, *Scientific Basis for the constitution in homoeopathy: <https://www.researchgate.net/publication/301204589_Scientific_Basis_for_the_Constitution_in_Homoeopathy>*

Vithoulkas, George 1980, *The science of homeopathy,* B. Jain Publishers, New Delhi.

Homoeopathic detoxification

Creedy, Melanie 2017, *High copper, environmental toxicity and thyroidinum,* <https://www.elementsofhealth.com.au/>.

Hubele, Lauren Feb, 2016, *Gemmotherapy, something to consider?* https://hpathy.com/homoeopathy-papers/>.

Hubele, Lauren June, 2018, *Dynamic gemmotherapy, beyond gemmotherapy, Volumes I and II,* <https://www.researchgate.net/publication/326048133_Dynamic_Gemmotherapy_Beyond_Gemmotherapy_Volumes_I_and_II>.

Maury, E.A. 1965, *Drainage in homoeopathy,* trans. Mark Clement, Health Science Press, Bradford, England.

McCall, Lee-Anne May, 2015, *CEASE therapy: a homoeopathic detoxification protocol,* <https://naturalmedicine.net.nz/news/cease-therapy-a-homoeopathic-detoxification-protocol/>.

Murphy, R n.d., *<http://www.lotushealthinstitute.com/articles/homeopathic-medicine-mainmenu-33/19-homeopathic-toxicology>.*

Smuts, Tinus Sep, 2017, *Autism treatment using homeopathy and isotherapy,* <https://aurumproject.org.au/autism-successful-treatment-using-homeopathy-and-isotherapy/>.

Swanson, Pamela, n.d.*Natural treatment for autism for children* in Florida, <https://homeopath-orlando.com/natural-treatments-for-children/natural-treatment-for-autism-for-children/>.

Tetau, Max n.d., *Organotherapy,* 2 vols, Brauer Biotherapies, Tanunda, South Australia.

Homoeopathic pharmacognosy

Chancellor, Philip M. 1971, *Illustrated handbook of the Bach flower remedies,* C.W. Daniel, Saffron Walden, Essex.

Murphy, R. 1995, *Lotus materia medica: homeopathic and spagyric medicines,* Lotus Star Academy, Pagosa Springs, Colorado.

Trease, G.E. and Evans, W.C. 1983, *Pharmacognosy,* 12th edn,. Balliere Tindall, London.

Twentyman, Ralph 1989, *The science and art of healing,* Floris Books, Edinburgh.

Verma, P.N. and Vaid, I. 1995, *Encyclopaedia of homoeopathic pharmacopoeia,* B. Jain Publishers, Delhi.

Weeks, Nora 1944, *The medical discoveries of Edward Bach, physician,* The C. W. Daniel Company Ltd, Saffron Walden, Essex.

Whitmont, Edward C. 1991, *Psyche and substance: essays on homeopathy in the light of Jungian psychology,* North Atlantic Books, Berkeley, California.

Homoeopathic pharmacy

Gaier, Harald C. 1991, *Thorsons encyclopaedic dictionary of homoeopathy: the definitive reference to all aspects of homoeopathy*, Thorsons, Hammersmith, London.

Kayne, Steven B. 1997, *Homoeopathic pharmacy: an introduction and handbook*, Churchill Livingstone, Edinburgh.

Isopathy

Gaier, Harald C. 1991, Thorsons encyclopaedic dictionary of homoeopathy: the definitive reference to all aspects of homoeopathy, Thorsons, Hammersmith, London.

Gurudas 1986, Gem elixirs and vibrational healing, vol 2, Cassandra Press, Boulder, Co.

Medhurst, Robert Jul, 2010, *Isopathy,* https://hpathy.com/homeopathy-papers/isopathy-2/.

Murphy, R. n.d., *Homeopath toxicology*, <http://www.alchemilla.com/articles/homeopathic-medicine-mainmenu-33/19-homeopathic-toxicology>.

Materia medica

Allen, H.C. n.d., *Keynotes with nosodes,* 8th edn, reprint, B. Jain Publishers, New Delhi.

Allen, H.C. n.d., *The materia medica of the nosodes with provings of the X-ray,* Jain Publishers, New Delhi.

Clarke, John Henry n.d., *A dictionary of practical materia medica,* 3 vols, Indian Books and Periodicals Syndicate, New Delhi.

Hahnemann, Samuel n.d., *Chronic diseases: their peculiar nature and their homoeopathic cure,* 2 vols, reprint, Indian Books and Periodicals Syndicate, New Delhi.

Hering, C. 1993, *The guiding symptoms of our materia medica,* reprint edn, 10 vols, B. Jain Publishers, New Delhi.

Kent, James Tyler 1911, *Lectures on homeopathic materia medica,* 2nd edn, Indian Books & Periodicals Syndicate, New Delhi.

Murphy, R. 1995, *Lotus materia medica: homeopathic and spagyric medicines,* Lotus Star Academy, Pagosa Springs, Colorado.

Nash, E.B. n.d., *Leaders in homeopathic therapeutics,* B. Jain Publishers, New Delhi.

Sankaran, Rajan 1992, *The spirit of homoeopathy,* 2nd edn, Homoeopathic Medical Publishers, Bombay.

Sankaran, Rajan 1994, *The substance of homoeopathy* 2nd edn, Homoeopathic Medical Publishers, Bombay.

Sankaran, Rajan 1997, *The soul of remedies,* Homoeopathic Medical Publishers, Bombay.

Scholten, Jan 1995, *Homoeopathy and minerals,* 2nd edn, Stichting Alonnissos, Utrecht.

Scholten, Jan 1996, *Homoeopathy and the elements,* Stichting Alonnissos, Utrecht.

Tyler, M. n.d., *Pointers to common remedies,* reprint, B. Jain Publishers, New Delhi.

Tyler, M.L. n.d., *Homoeopathic drug pictures* 2nd edn, reprint, B. Jain Publishers, New Delhi.

Verma, P.N. and Vaid, I. 1995, *Encyclopaedia of homoeopathic pharmacopoeia,* B. Jain Publishers, Delhi.

Vermeulen, F. 1994, *Concordant materia medica,* Merlijn Publishers, Haarlem, Netherlands.

Miasms

Choudhary, Harimohan 1997, *Indications of miasm,* B. Jain Publishers, New Delhi.

Koehler, Gerhard 1986, *The handbook of homoeopathy: its principles and practice,* trans. A.R. Meuss, Thorsons Publishing Group, Wellingborough, Northamptonshire.

Murphy, R. n.d., Miasms chart, <http://www.lotushealthinstitute.com/articles/homeopathic-medicine-mainmenu-33/17-miasms-chart>.

Ortega, Proceso S. 1980, *Notes on the miasms, trans.* Harris Coulter, National homoeopathic Pharmacy, New Delhi.

Speight, P.A. 1977, *Comparison of the chronic miasms, rev.,* Health Science Press, Saffron Walden, Essex, England.

New physics

Bateson, Gregory 1980, *Mind and nature: a necessary unity,* Bantam Books, Toronto.

Blair, Lawrence 1976, *Rhythms of vision: the changing patterns of belief,* Paladin, Frogmore, St Albans, Herts.

Bohm, David 1981, *Wholeness and the implicate order,* Routledge and Kegan Paul, London.

Bohm, David 1985, *Unfolding meaning: a weekend of dialogue with David Bohm,* Ark Paperbacks, London.

Chalmers, A.F. 1976, *What is this thing called science? An assessment of the nature and status of science and its methods,* University of Queensland Press, St Lucia.

Coates Callum 1996, *Living energies: an exposition of concepts related to the theories of Viktor Schauberger,* Gateway Books, Bath, UK.

Eisenstein, Charles, n.d., *The impact of morphic resonance,* <https://uplift.love/the-impact-of-morphic-resonance/>.

Martin, Y., n.d., *Morphic field and morphic resonance,* <https://www.spiritualresources.info/morphic-fieldresonance>.

Pawlicki, T.B. 1984, *How you can explore higher dimensions of space and time,* Prentice-Hall, Englewood Cliffs, New Jersey.

Percival, Harold W. 1974, *Thinking and destiny,* The Word Foundation Inc, Dallas, Texas.

Sheldrake, R. 1985, *A new science of life: The hypothesis of formative causation*, 2nd ed, Anthony Blond, London.

Sheldrake, R. 2009, *Morphic resonance: the nature of formative causation,* 4th rev. and expanded U.S. edn, Park Street Press, Rochester, Vermont.

Sheldrake R., n.d., *Morphic resonance and morphic fields - an introduction,* <https://www.sheldrake.org/research/morphic-resonance/introduction>.

Sheldrake R.,Spring, 1987, *Part 1 - Mind, memory and archetype: morphic resonance and the collective unconscious,* <https://www.sheldrake.org/research/morphic-resonance/part-1-mind-memory-and-archetype-morphic-resonance-and-the-collective-unconscious>.

Talbot, Michael 1991, *The holographic universe,* HarperPerennial, NY.

Teilhard de Chardin, Pierre 1965, *The phenomenon of man,* Collins Fontana Books, London.

Thompson, Eric, n.d., *Morphic resonance: an introduction to biofield science part 1,* <http://www.iawaketechnologies.com/morphic-resonance/>.

Toben, Bob and Wolf, Fred Alan 1982, *Space-time and beyond,* E.P. Dutton, New York.

Wilber, Ken (ed) 1982, *The holographic paradigm and other paradoxes: exploring the leading edge of science,* Shambhala, Boulder, Colorado.

Wilber, Ken 1990, *Eye to eye: the quest for the new paradigm,* expanded edn, Shambhala, Boston, Massachusetts.

Wolf, Fred Alan 1987, *The body quantum: the new physics of body, mind and health*. Heinemann, London.

Non-standard homoeopathics

Chancellor, Philip M 1971, *Illustrated handbook of the Bach flower remedies,* C.W. Daniel, Saffron Walden, Essex.

Tansley, David 1972, *Radionics and the subtle anatomy of man,* Health Science Press, London.

Tansley, David V. 1975, *Radionics: interface with the ether fields,* The C.W. Daniel Company Ltd, Saffron Walden, Essex, England.

Tansley, David 1977, *Subtle body: essence and shadow,* Thames and Hudson, London.

Tansley, David V. 1992, *Dimensions of radionics: techniques of instrumented distant healing,* Brotherhood of Life, Inc., Albuquerque, New Mexico.

Tetau Max n.d.. *Gemmotherapy*, Dolisos, Paris.

Tyler, Gina Apr, 2007, *Homeopathy and radiaesthesia,* <https://hpathy.com/homeopathy-papers/homeopathy-and-radiaesthesia/>.

Vlamis, Gregory 1990, *Flower remedies to the rescue: the healing vision of Dr Edward Bach,* Thorsons Publishing Group, Wellingborough, Northamptonshire, England.

Weeks, Nora 1944, *The medical discoveries of Edward Bach, physician,* The C. W. Daniel Company Ltd, Saffron Walden, Essex.

White, Ian 1991, *Australian bush flower essences,* Bantam Books, Sydney.

Obstacles to cure

Field, Robert Apr 2018., *Obstacles to cure,* <https://www.homeobook.com/obstacle-to-cure-the-principles-and-art-of-cure-by-homoeopathy-by-ha-robert>.

Poole, Jennifer Jan, 2017, *Establishing a scientific foundation in homeopathy:* <https://www.researchgate.net/publication/314606983_Establishing_a_Scientific_Foundation_for_Homeopath_2_Identifying_and_treating_maintaining_causes>.

Potency and posology

Choudhary, H. 1990, *50 millesimal potency in theory and practice,* 3rd edn, B. Jain Publishers, New Delhi.
Dhawale, M.L. 1985, *Principles and practice of homoeopathy,* 2nd edn, Institute of Clinical Research, Bombay.
Gaier, Harald C. 1991, *Thorsons encyclopaedic dictionary of homoeopathy: the definitive reference to all aspects of homoeopathy,* Thorsons, Hammersmith, London.
Hahnemann, Samuel 1842, *Organon of the medical art,* 6th edn, ed. and annot. Wenda Brewster O'Reilly, trans. Stephen Decker, Birdcage Books, Redmond, Washington.
Kent, James Tyler n.d., *Lectures on homoeopathic philosophy, reprint,* B. Jain Publishers, New Delhi.
Lessell, Colin B. 1994, *The infinitesimal dose: the scientific roots of homoeopathy,* The C.W. Daniel Company Ltd, Saffron Walden.
Morgan, John Jan, 2012, *Dose, dilution and the LM potencies,* <https://hpathy.com/homeopathy-papers/dose-dilution-and-the-lm-potencies/>.
Murphy, Robin 1994, *Organon philosophy workbook,* HANA, Pagosa Springs, Colorado.
Rafeeque, M. Feb, 2016, *An insight into LM potencies and divided doses,* <https://hpathy.com/homeopathy-papers/insight-into-lm-potencies/>.
Tyler, Gina Apr, 2007, *Homeopathy and radiaesthesia,* <https://hpathy.com/homeopathy-papers/homeopathy-and-radiaesthesia/>.
Vithoulkas, George 1980, *The science of homoeopathy,* B. Jain Publishers, New Delhi.

Prophylaxis

Julian, O.A. 1985, *Treatise on dynamised immunotherapy,* 2nd edn, B. Jain Publishers, New Delhi.

Thomson, K. and Miksevicius, E. 1988, *Vaccination: research, information and guidelines for homoeopathic practitioners,* Australian Institute of Homoeopathy, Sydney.

Whatcott, Cilla Apr, 2017, *Homoeoprophylaxis in India,* <https://www.westonaprice.org/health-topics/homeopathy/homeoprophylaxis-in-india>.

Proving

Doré, David Nov, 2012, *Provings,* <https://hpathy.com/homeopathy-papers/provings/>.

Gaier, Harald C. 1991, *Thorsons encyclopaedic dictionary of homoeopathy: the definitive reference to all aspects of homoeopathy,* Thorsons, Hammersmith, London.

Kayne, Steven B. 1997, *Homoeopathic pharmacy: an introduction and handbook,* Churchill Livingstone, Edinburgh.

Sherr, J. 1994, *The dynamics and methodology of homoeopathic provings,* Dynamis Books, Malvern, Worcs., UK.

Vithoulkas, George 1980, *The science of homoeopathy,* B. Jain Publishers, New Delhi.

Repertory

Clarke, John Henry n.d., *A clinical repertory to the dictionary of materia medica,* Indian Books and Periodicals Syndicate, New Delhi.

Murphy, R. 1996, *Homeopathic medical repertory,* 2nd edn, Hahnemann Academy of North America, Durango, Colorado.

Schroyens, F. 1995, *Synthesis,* Homoeopathic Book Publishers, London.

Research into homoeopathy

Bellavite, P. and Signorini, A. 1995, *Homoeopathy: a frontier in medical science,* North Atlantic Books, Berkeley, California.

Results analysis and second prescription

Dhawale, M.L. 1985, *Principles and practice of homoeopathy,* 2nd edn, Institute of Clinical Research, Bombay.

Cazalet, S 1999, *The second prescription by James Tyler Kent,* <http://homeoint.org/cazalet/kent/secondpre.htm>.

Schuett, Katja Jun, 2013, *Aggravation in homoeopathy,* <https://hpathy.com/organon-philosophy/aggravation-in-homeopathy/>.

Vithoulkas, George 1980, *The science of homoeopathy,* B. Jain Publishers, New Delhi.

Terminal illness

Bello, Lia Jan, 2017, *End of life care - homoeopathy and hospice patients,* <https://hpathy.com/homeopathy-papers/end-of-life-care-homeopathy-and-hospice-patients>.

DiPasquale, Robin Jun, 2012, *A place for plants in conscious end of life,* https://ndnr.com/botanical-medicine/a-place-for-plants-in-conscious-end-of-life.

Muttathukunnel, Paul 2017, *Palliative homoeopathic treatment in advanced cancer cases,* https://www.homeopathy360.com/2017/03/16/palliative-homeopathic-treatment-in-advanced-cancer-cases.

Smith, Sue Apr, 2015, *The end of life and homeopathy,* <https://hpathy.com/homeopathy-papers/the-end-of-life-and-homeopathy>.

Theory and philosophy of homoeopathy

Allan, N. n.d., *Beyond substance,* http://www.normanallan.com/Sci/bs.html.

Blackie, Margery Grace 1990, *Classical homoeopathy,* Charles Elliot and Frank Johnson (eds), Beaconsfield Publishers, Beaconsfield, Bucks.

Borland, Douglass M. 1982, *Homoeopathy in practice,* ed. Kathleen Priestman, Keats Publishing, New Canaan, Connecticut.

Close, Stuart n.d., *The genius of homoeopathy: lectures and essays on homoeopathic philosophy,* reprint, B. Jain Publishers, New Delhi.

Clover, Anne 1989, *Homoeopathy reconsidered: a new look at Hahnemann's Organon,* Victor Gollancz, London.

Coulter, Harris L. 1980, *Homeopathic science and modern medicine: the physics of healing with microdoses,* North Atlantic Books, Berkeley, California.

Dhawale, M.L. 1985, *Principles and practice of homoeopathy,* 2nd edn, Institute of Clinical Research, Bombay.

Dudgeon, R.E. 1994, *Lectures on the theory and practice of homoeopathy,* B. Jain Publishers, New Delhi.

Gaier, Harald C. 1991, *Thorsons encyclopaedic dictionary of homoeopathy: the definitive reference to all aspects of homoeopathy,* Thorsons, Hammersmith, London.

Hahnemann, Samuel 1842, *Organon of the medical art,* 6th edn, ed. and annot. Wenda Brewster O'Reilly, trans. Stephen Decker, Birdcage Books, Redmond, Washington.

Hahnemann, Samuel n.d., *Lesser Writings,* ed. and trans. R.E. Dudgeon, reprint, B. Jain Publishers, New Delhi.

Handley, Rima 1987, *Classical Hahnemannian homoeopathy or What Hahnemann really did: preliminary observations,* quoted in Gaier, *op. cit., p. 98.*

Handley, Rima 1997, *In search of the later Hahnemann,* Beaconsfield Homoeopathic Library, Beaconsfield, Bucks, UK.

Hubbard, Elizabeth Wright 1990, *Homoeopathy as art and science,* Maesimund Panos and Della DesRosiers (eds), Beaconsfield Publishers Ltd, Beaconsfield, Bucks, England.

Jefferies, Helen, Welch, Elle & Santiago, Paloma Vazquez Jul, 2013, *Susceptibility,* <https://hpathy.com/organon-philosophy/susceptibility-2/>.

Kent, James Tyler n.d., *Lectures on homoeopathic philosophy, reprint,* B. Jain Publishers, New Delhi.

Koehler, Gerhard 1986, *The handbook of homoeopathy: its principles and practice,* trans. A.R. Meuss, Thorsons Publishing Group, Wellingborough, Northamptonshire.

Morell, Peter, undated, Review of Handley, Rima, 1007: *In search of the later Hahnemann,* <http://www.homoeoint.org/morrell/articles/pm_rima.htm.

Murphy, Robin 1994, *Organon philosophy workbook,* HANA, Pagosa Springs, Colorado.

Norland, Misha Oct, 2009, *Susceptibility,* <https://hpathy.com/organon-philosophy/susceptibility>.

Roberts, Herbert A. 1985, *The principles and art of cure by homoeopathy,* B. Jain Publishers, New Delhi.

Sangupta, D. Aug, 2015, *Concepts of homoeopathy with its principles, doctrines and laws: co-relation with modern views,* <https://hpathy.com/organon-philosophy/concepts-of-homoeopathy-with-its-principles-doctrines-and-laws-co-relation-with-modern-views/>.

Speight, Phyllis 1979, *A study course in homoeopathy,* Health Science Press, Bradford.

Twentyman, Ralph 1989, *The science and art of healing,* Floris Books, Edinburgh.

Vithoulkas, George 1980, *The science of homoeopathy,* B. Jain Publishers, New Delhi.

Therapeutics

Fisher, Leslie 1993, *The clinical science of mineral therapy,* The Maurice Blackmore Research Foundation, Balgowlah, NSW.

Gilbert, Peter 1989, *Mineral tissue salts,* Thorsons Publishing Group, Wellingborough, Northamptonshire.

Jouanny, Jaques 1994, *The essentials of homoeopathic therapeutics,* Boirons, S.A., France.

Hughes, Richard 1997, *The principles and practice of homoeopathy, reprint,* B. Jain Publishers, New Delhi.

Kichlu, K. and Bose, L. 1979, *Descriptive medicine,* 2nd edn, B. Jain Publishers, New Delhi.

Lilienthal, S. 1925, *Homoeopathic therapeutics,* B. Jain Publishers, New Delhi.

Lockie, Andrew 1990, *The family guide to homoeopathy: the safe form of medicine for the future,* Hamish Hamilton, London.

Logan, Robin 1988, *The homoeopathic treatment of eczema,* Beaconsfield Publishers, Beaconsfield.

Mathur, Kaylash Narayan 1975, *Principles of prescribing,* B. Jain Publishers, New Delhi.

Moskowitz, Richard 1992, *Homeopathic medicines for pregnancy and childbirth,* North Atlantic Books, Berkeley, California.

Smuts, Tinus Sep, 2017, *Autism treatment using homeopathy and isotherapy,* <https://aurumproject.org.au/autism-successful-treatment-using-homeopathy-and-isotherapy/>.

Tissue salts

Fisher, Leslie 1993, *The clinical science of mineral therapy,* The Maurice Blackmore Research Foundation, Balgowlah, NSW.

Gilbert, Peter 1989, *Mineral tissue salts,* Thorsons Publishing Group, Wellingborough, Northamptonshire.

Lessell, Colin B. 1984, *The biochemic handbook,* rev., Thorsons Publishing Group, Wellingborough, Northamptonshire.

Vaccination

Australian Vaccination Network 1988, *Vaccination roulette: experiences, risks and alternatives,* AVN, Bangalow, NSW.

Miller, Neil Z. 1994, *Vaccines: are they really safe and effective?: A parent's guide to childhood shots,* rev., New Atlantean Press, Santa Fe, New Mexico.

Scheibner, Vera 1993, *Vaccination,* Blackheath, NSW.

Sinclair, Ian 1992, *Vaccination: the hidden facts,* Wagaman, NT.

Vitalistic medicine

Barasch, Marc Ian 1995, *The healing path: a soul approach to illness,* Penguin Arkana, New York.

Bek, Lilla and Pullar, Philippa 1986, *The seven levels of healing,* Rider, London.

Davidson, John 1988, *The web of life: life force—the energetic constitution of man and the neuro-endocrine connection,* The C.W. Daniel Company Limited, Saffron Walden.

Dethlefsen, Thorwald 1989, *The challenge of fate,* trans. Eva M. Loewe and Christopher McIntosh, Coventure, Boston.

Dethlefsen, Thorwald and Dahlke, Rüdiger 1990, *The healing power of illness: the meaning of symptoms and how to interpret them,* trans. Peter Lemesurier, Element Books, Longmead, Shaftesbury, Dorset.

Dossey, Larry 1982, *Space, time and medicine,* Shambhala, Boulder.

Gerber, Richard 1988, *Vibrational medicine: new choices for healing ourselves,* Bear and Co., Santa Fe, NM.

Grossinger, Richard 1990, *Planet medicine: from stone age shamanism to post-industrial healing,* 5th edn, North Atlantic Books, Berkeley, California.

Harrison, John 1984, *Love your disease: it's keeping you healthy,* Angus and Robertson, North Ryde.
Howard, W. 2005, *Vitalism revitalised,* <http://www.smeddum.net/articles/vitalism.htm>.
Levine, Stephen 1989, *Healing into life and death,* Gateway Books, Bath.
Schaef, Anne Wilson 1992, *Beyond therapy, beyond science: a new model for healing the whole person,* Harper, San Francisco.
Whitmont, Edward C. 1991, *Psyche and substance: essays on homeopathy in the light of Jungian psychology,* North Atlantic Books, Berkeley, California.
Whitmont, Edward C. 1993, *The Alchemy of healing: Psyche and soma,* North Atlantic Books, Berkeley, California.
Whitmont, Ronald D. Apr, 2011, *Psychosomatics and homeopathy,* <https://www.homoeopathicmd.com/2011/04>.
Wood, Matthew 1992, *The magical staff: the vitalist tradition in western medicine,* North Atlantic Books, Berkeley, California.

About the author

Peter Twohig BA, BA (Hons), BHlthSc (Hom), DHeal, ND (Adv), DBotMed, DNut, DHom, DAIHom, GrDHomMed

Former Director:
Littlewood Clinic of Homoeopathic and Energistic Medicine

Former Principal:
Armstrong College of Natural Medicine
College of the Australian Institute of Homoeopathy

Former Senior Lecturer:
Endeavour College of Natural Health

Former Lecturer:
College of the International Yoga Teachers Association
Nature Care College of Natural & Traditional Medicine
Unity College of Healing

Prior to practising medicine, Peter had a career in management consulting and computer system development. Peter's career in healing began when he became a Reiki channel. He eventually met channels who also worked in other fields, and was introduced to homoeopathy, naturopathy, neurolinguistic programming (NLP), past life therapy, and psychic healing.

He has since given up his medical practice in order to concentrate on writing. Peter is also an award-winning fiction writer and poet. He comes from Melbourne, but now lives in sunny Gosford, on the New South Wales Central Coast, and is interested in, well, everything.

Drop into my website:

WildHomoeopathy.com, where you'll find a blog, and lots of further reading and news of projected works.

BOOKS BY PETER

LITERARY FICTION

The Richmond Trilogy

The Cartographer
The Torch
The Mazemaster (Out in 2021)

Other novels

An Ill-fitting Man (Out in 2021)

SCIENCE FICTION

The Messiah Trilogy

The Last Messiah (Out in 2022)

BOOKS FOR HOMOEOPATHS

A Vitalistic Approach to Homoeopathic Medicine
Case Management as a Clinical Technology
Introduction to Isopathic Prescribing
The Homoeopathic Approach to Autism (Out in 2021)

The Homoeopathy 2.0 Series

Homoeopathy is undergoing a rebirth. At the same time, a world-wide explosion of interest in alternative medicine and healing technologies is taking place. In the spirit of this movement, the Homoeopathy 2.0 series of books has arrived.

The complete Homoeopathy 2.0 series of three books will:

- provide you with a deeper understanding of the philosophy of homoeopathy, thereby diminishing its mystique
- reveal a multitude of ways to use potentialised medicines, both singly and in combination to achieve results
- offer modern and common-sense formulations of homoeopathic concepts that can be used to adopt sound and logical prescribing habits
- show you how to bring to bear a battery of prescribing techniques and theories to help you create a more confident clinical practice
- recontextualise your training and experience within a vitalistic framework, thus enabling you to reconnect with a workable classical view
- explain why potencies behave the way they do, and how to use that knowledge in the clinic.
- clarify vague concepts of, for example, potency election, constitutional remedies, detoxification, miasms, antidoting, aggravation, and prophylaxis supply you with the means to deal with the issues of modern homoeopathy once and for all.

Book 1 - A Vitalistic Approach to Homoeopathic Medicine

This book provides:

- an outline of the principles of vitalistic medicine as they relate to homoeopathy
- a revised homoeopathic pharmacodynamic system
- a revision, along classical lines, of homoeopathic theory, and an outline of its clinical applications.

Book 2 - Case Management as a Clinical Technology

This book provides:

- an implementation of the principles enunciated in Book 1 specially designed to achieve improved results in cases of chronic disease
- case analysis, repertorising, and potency and dosage selection advice from the first consultation to the final review
- strategies and therapeutic guidelines for the management of notoriously difficult classes of case.

Book 3 - Introduction to Isopathic Prescribing

This book provides:

- a theory of group disease (including its displacement of miasmic theory)
- an introduction to the principles of isopathic technology using potentised remedies
- strategies and therapeutic guidelines for the management of detoxification
- strategies and therapeutic guidelines for the management of prophylaxis
- a set of palliative protocols for treating certain categories of commonly seen disorders.

Made in the USA
Las Vegas, NV
23 March 2026

44120322R00122